SIX WEEKS TO OMG

VENICE A. FULTON

SIX WEEKS TO OMG

GET SKINNIER THAN ALL YOUR FRIENDS

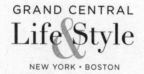

GRAND CENTRAL
Life & Style

NEW YORK · BOSTON

Neither this nor any other diet and exercise program should be followed without first consulting a health care professional. If you have any special conditions requiring attention, you should consult with your health care professional regularly regarding possible modification of the program contained in this book.

Grand Central Life & Style
Hachette Book Group
237 Park Avenue
New York, NY 10017

www.HachetteBookGroup.com

Printed in the United States of America

RRD-C

First Edition: July 2012
10 9 8 7 6 5 4 3 2 1

Grand Central Life & Style is an imprint of Grand Central Publishing. The Grand Central Life & Style name and logo are trademarks of Hachette Book Group, Inc.

The Hachette Speakers Bureau provides a wide range of authors for speaking events. To find out more, go to www.HachetteSpeakersBureau.com or call (866) 376-6591.

The publisher is not responsible for websites (or their content) that are not owned by the publisher.

Library of Congress Control Number: 2012940408

DYING IS THE WRONG OMG

SEE YOUR DOCTOR BEFORE YOU DIET

For Bella,

Who is everything that's beautiful in life, all at once.

You, and no one else, make me feel like anything is possible.

I love you very much.

TURNING PAGES BURNS FAT

AND THE OSCAR GOES TO…

YOU!

Dear reader, this section of a book is normally called the 'Acknowledgements'. It's such a long word. I mean, why bother when nobody usually reads that part! But this time, I hope you'll make an exception, because I want to thank *you*.

Without you, this book wouldn't exist. This really *is* sounding like an Oscar speech! But it's true, without people who want to improve something, our planet would just stay the same. Making things better is what keeps the human race going.

And perhaps the greatest something to improve, is ourselves. It takes guts to admit that things aren't perfect, and it takes even more guts to do something about it. Most people talk big, and act small. You're already braver and smarter than them.

Sometimes there are naughty types who sense your dream to find a better way, and they take advantage. I saw this happen way too often, and like you, I decided to make things better. I wrote this book. And now, I'm going to get you that first OMG.

Venice A. Fulton

London, England

January 1, 2012

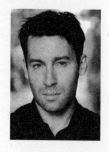

CUT THE CRAP

The medical community think you shouldn't read this book. Your parents might think you shouldn't read this book. Perhaps even your friends think you shouldn't read this book. And you're still reading?

Good job! It's your life. Only you walk around in your shoes. Only you wake up with your thoughts. And only you will fall asleep to them. *Should* and *shouldn't* are useless words. Even reading them can make you feel under pressure. Trash them!

KNOWLEDGE IS GOLDEN

Before this book hit the mainstream, it came under lots of fire. With *OMG* and *Skinny* in the title, I suppose it was to be expected. What I didn't expect, was criticism from those who hadn't actually read it. That's like criticizing your blind date *before* they show up!

Scientists are taught to *not* do that (in a metaphorical sense of course, as scientists don't go on dates), but sometimes even they slip up. We live in a world full of information, and to prevent overload, we often dismiss huge chunks of it in a heartbeat.

When it comes to your health, I urge you to criticize *nothing* without good reason. There's just a chance that beyond all the smiles, and jokey comments, there's some jaw-dropping science waiting to help you. I didn't invent it, or even discover it. I simply didn't *dismiss* it. Be open, be open, be open.

The only way to *truly* silence people is to show them what you mean. If you live this book for 6 weeks, you'll do that. And if you change as much as I know you can, they'll be surprised enough to greet new you with those 3 magic letters, 'O – M – G'!

Many industry people worried when they found out I was going to write this. Why? Because they knew I'd cut the crap. And they knew that if I did that, you'd probably stop buying their next diet, exercise 'secret', or food product.

I believe that if you simply get *told* to do something, you'll stick to it for a while, and succeed, for a while. And that's the problem. After you stop getting told, you just rebel and slowly go back to what you're used to.

I also know that when you *understand* how stuff works, you'll stick to it. In fact when you really understand, it won't feel like you need to stick to it at all. You'll simply stop thinking about those old habits and old beliefs, and you'll have developed new mechanisms. **Permanent success!**

WHY ARE YOU READING THAT?

Many will say that you don't need any help, including parents. They might state that, 'you're fine as you are', 'it's unhealthy', or repeat the classic, 'it's just puppy fat'. Guess what, YOU'RE NOT A PUPPY! Are they right about the other stuff?

No. Only you can ever decide if you're *fine*. No one else. Even with serious eating disorders, bad habits only stop when a patient changes how *they* see themselves. As early as you can, develop the skill of seeing yourself accurately.

Is this book unhealthy? No. I can hear doctors muttering in the distance! If you're young, they believe you *should* just let Mother Nature take care of things. If 'Mom knows best', Mom Nature can surely be left alone, and all be okay.

Yeah right! Allowed to be natural, we can order pizza at midnight or travel miles without hardly moving a muscle. We live in a world full of modern luxuries. Mother Nature left town 30 years ago and she's not coming back!

Doctors are very aware of research that shows most adult diseases usually start when we're young, and are linked to being too fat. They also know that if you stay skinny when you're young, you're less likely to be a fadult (a fat adult).

Despite knowing this, the medical community is always very sensible. They think it's best to *play it safe*. It's dangerous to play it safe! It's much more sensible to start taking a big interest in yourself, by learning about what works today.

This book will also boost your mental health by helping you look good and feel more in control. Having confidence is crucial, and getting it today is tougher than at any time in human history. You deserve to walk with confidence **now**.

What about the media? They're pretty hard on you. On the one hand, they fill pages and screens with beautiful people who look totally amazing all year round. It's no surprise; beautiful people sell lots of magazines, TV shows and movies.

What is a surprise is when the same shows or magazines criticize *you* for trying to be the same. Talk about confusing. The media is in the business of selling stuff, so when it comes to their fast opinions and nasty news articles, forgetaboutit!

Now, this is a tough one. Friends. Maybe you're secretly in competition with some? Hey, maybe they're secretly in competition with you! I just want you to realize something about friends. It applies to people you might work with too.

They're scared. Not jealous, *scared*. Applying this book could rocket you to happiness and they don't want to be left behind. Of course they could do the same, but we humans seem to think that only one person can be successful at a time!

Because of that fear, don't expect them to help you. Some might even go too far and discourage you. Now, I'm not telling you to ignore your friends completely. We need friends. I mean who else are we going to show off to!

"IT'S ALL ABOUT YOU, ISN'T IT?"

Yes it is, actually! And why not? If there's one thing I'd love you to take away from reading this book, it's a new found respect for *you*. Hold on for a second, don't just skip past that sentence because your brain has heard it before.

Respect yourself. I mean it. I'm not heading down the cliché known as, "if you don't respect yourself, who will?". That's not relevant! You need to respect yourself, fully and always make the smartest decisions.

Destiny sounds mystical and romantic, but it's nothing more than a whole bunch of decisions made back to back. In an ideal world, you make brilliant decision after brilliant decision. Of course, sometimes it's not an ideal world.

The great thing is, a few tiny wrong turns *can* be corrected. How? Shut your eyes (not recommended if you're walking or driving), breathe normally, be honest, and wait for your heart to speak up. It's always right. Always.

When you lose hope in this book, and feel like ripping it up, stop. Go to the store, and rip up *other* diet books! Seriously, take a moment, and ask yourself if you've been honest with your actions. If you really have, please rip this up too, and move on.

The take home message is this: **be relentless in your pursuit of happy-ness**. The quality of your life is simply down to what *feelings* you have most often throughout the moment, minute, hour, day, week, month, year, decade, ta-da, *life*.

No one cares more about you, than you. No one lives in your mind or body, but you. The person in the mirror, that's you. Absolutely everything is down, to you. And, when those OMG reactions start flying your way, only you can say, *I did that*.

HOW TO GET THE SKINNY ON

To get the best out of this book, and that means to get the best out of you, it's good to read it at a time when you can fully concentrate. You will boost your success when you really know *how* stuff works, instead of just doing what I say.

Take a few days to read it. If it's not starting to click, find a different chair, bed or beanbag, and read it again! I want you to become an expert. Experts don't just read a summary or listen to someone who 'did that diet'. An expert *gets it.*

Each technique is written so that you can try it by itself and see what effect it has (and see if you can handle it!). But I can tell you now, when you use all the techniques at the same time, your progress will be become much faster.

This happens because even though your body appears as one object, it's made up of a ridiculously huge amount of parts. The spares catalogue for one human body would fill an entire library! When all the parts talk to each other, we really fly.

At the end of each section, I'll repeat 6 OMG-getting facts to help you *get the skinny on* whatever's just been said (plus 1 simple bit of take-out advice). I may seem to repeat myself (it's deliberate). Don't rely on these sum-ups only!

And just one more thing; I'm assuming that you're not suffering from a medical condition or need medication before you start. Being overweight is unhealthy, but for some, any change in routine could be unhealthy too. Be smart.

If you're worried, ask your doctor or health professional to read this. Don't let them make a snap judgment by skimming through it, or worse, getting *you* to explain it. Lots of doctors could actually learn something from reading it. Am I joking?

Nope. Medical students spend little time on diet or health, often less than 1 day from 5 years of studying. Doctors are trained to *discover and treat disease*, and not to *improve health*. And they know absolutely nothing about getting you OMGs!

This book uses very plain English, and paragraph spacing that annoys those who make formatting rules. I don't care about rules. I care about you *getting it*, and that's why you see what you see. Fancy graphics or pictures are for comics. You just need the truth.

Before we go further, I need you to do something for me. **Keep an open mind**. At one time, most people believed that the world was flat, and that if you went too far, you'd *fall* off. Be a brave captain, it's time to set sail.

GET THE SKINNY ON...

OMG 6 Only read when you can think straight

OMG 5 Keep reading until it all clicks

OMG 4 The key to success is understanding stuff

OMG 3 If you don't get it, keep going until you do

OMG 2 If you see doctors or take meds, ask them about doing this diet

OMG 1 Keep an open mind about what you'll find in the book

OMG ! Don't just rely on these summaries!

HIGH FIVE

If you really want to know how-to-wow in a hurry, you've got to attack certain key problems. Beauty is in the eye of the beholder, but it seems that there are **5 main areas** which most people want to focus on. These become our basic goals:

1 – LOSE FAT

I know, obvious. But it's important to state it. More than anything, carrying too much fat is the thing that upsets most people in terms of appearance. It's easy to get fat these days, but with modern fashion and pressures, it's not easy to hide.

The majority of this book will focus on getting rid of this unwanted fat. From a scientific point of view, it makes sense. When you take care of what's making you fat, your body starts improving all your other problem areas.

To make sure that you lose fat permanently, I'm going to tell you the truth like you've never heard it. Once you really understand how the body wants to play, you'll keep it off easily. And best of all, you can *start* to stop thinking about this stuff!

2 – GET TONED

When you lose fat, your skin moves closer to your muscles, and in some ways you'll appear more toned. Hold on though, that's just how you *look*. To get properly toned, that's throughout your whole body, you need to do something for it.

If you don't do that, and someone gets close enough to touch test your success, you might still feel as soft as a marshmallow! Some people are naturally more toned than others, but even they would benefit from specific help.

Developing a firm feeling body will actually give you an inner confidence, one that's just a squeeze away. How? Feeling your own toned muscles will remind you that there's a body within, full of potential. It's your built-in trainer!

The techniques used for getting toned will also benefit your general health. Being toned isn't just for some people. We can all 'be like that'. And when you are, you'll have a body that doesn't just look like it works, it really *will* work.

3 – SLIM DOWN YOUR THIGHS

Skirts, skinny jeans, hot pants, summer dresses. It seems that the fashion industry is obsessed with putting pins on show! With so much media and social emphasis put on female thighs, it's no surprise that improving them comes high on your list.

Apparently, you want them thinner, firmer, smoother and without cellulite. Oh, and you also wouldn't mind them being a bit longer! I can deal with pretty much all of those (yes even the last one, because slimmer legs always look longer).

Normally, I'd say run a mile if a health expert says that they've got a 'secret'. But, I have something that's so unusual, so rarely used, and so effective, that it actually deserves to be called a secret. Your thighs and eyes will love it.

4 – FLATTEN YOUR BELLY

Having a toned and flat middle never used to be that important. Then came belly rings, short tops, and modern fabrics so thin that nothing is left to the imagination! If you want to feel good today, it's impossible to ignore the middle of your body.

Our middle is where we keep our feelings, it's there when we stand, when we lie down, and it even says 'HELLO' when we sit down! You can hide your tummy from others, but it's got a cheeky habit of following you around.

Scientists have discovered that a flatter belly isn't just a sexy look. It's proof that you're getting lots of things right. This also means that even if you're skillful at hiding a big belly in clothes, you can't hide its affect on your health.

5 - KEEP YOUR SKIN, HAIR AND NAILS GLOWING

Although these areas weren't my first thoughts when writing this book, it became obvious to me that you can't get an OMG reaction if your skin and hair look awful. Many diet and health books don't think about skin and hair. Do you?

Programs often work on some areas while skin, hair and nails slowly suffer in the background. Many assume that it's a price we have to pay. Rubbish! Our skin is our largest organ, and if it's suffering, something's not right.

Our hair, like our skin, also gives us clues about how healthy we really are, i.e. on the inside. Expensive skin creams and hair products are fun, but they can't fix deeper problems. Everything you get from me will benefit your beauty bits.

You can do this. All five. And when you do, I'm certain that you'll feel amazing. Even better, you'll be back in control.

Back in control? Yes, back in control. If you're reading this, there's probably a part of you that feels things have gotten out of control. When people feel powerless for too long, it can turn into 'what's the point?'. That's a truly dangerous sentence.

I can't tell you what your ultimate goal is. It's *personal*. But I definitely know that when you get in control of your body and health, your mind becomes free to be brilliant in whatever way you want. Come on, let's turn the page!

GET THE SKINNY ON...

OMG 6 You will lose fat

OMG 5 You will get toned all over

OMG 4 You will slim down your thighs

OMG 3 You will flatten your belly

OMG 2 You will have lovely hair, skin and nails

OMG 1 You will feel good about yourself

OMG ! You will get back in control if you turn the page!

HOW, HOW, HOW

'How fat do you think I am?'

'How much do you think I can lose?'

'How quickly do you think I could lose it?'

HOW FAT DO YOU THINK I AM?

Outside of a book, you might have asked this as 'do you think I'm fat?'. Some of you have an answer already, and some of you could even be right. The majority won't be. By the end of the section, you'll have much more confidence in the truth.

For many, this question is important because it leads onto the next ('how much do you think I can lose?'). You usually want an *exact* answer. Maybe you've already been given one from someone else. Here's the news. Listen to no one!

Everyone has opinions. Friends offer advice in blocks of five, 'you need to lose 10lbs / 15lbs / 20lbs'! A doctor will use charts, a formula, or technical sounding words. And a parent might just say 'lots'!

FRIENDS AND FAMILY

The people you see often will definitely have strong opinions about how you look. But being close doesn't automatically make them an expert. If anything, it makes them less likely to come up with an accurate answer.

Parents may negatively (or positively) compare you to a brother, sister, relation, or even themselves. This is wrong. Even within families, genetics and habits vary, making these opinions simplistic.

For the same reason, the viewpoint of a close friend may also not be of much use. And there's always a chance they could feel threatened by giving you an honest answer, and watching your success as they feel left behind.

DOCTORS

Doctors are widely trusted to be experts on our health. As I've said already, they're actually experts at disease. A doctor studies for 5 years or more, but they only spend a day on diet. Better hope *they* weren't sick that day!

If you ask Doc for help, they'll be limited to using a few standard techniques. Firstly, they'll weigh you. I'll talk about weighing later, but right now, the scales aren't important. It's how a doctor uses them.

After reading your weight, a doctor will usually do one or two things. They'll get out a chart, they'll ask you for your height, and finally, if they're feeling very scientific, they'll bring out their secret weapon: the calculator!

HEIGHT AND WEIGHT TABLES

If your doctor shows you one of these, it says they're *old school*. Height and weight charts were designed in the 1950s to help a big insurance company decide if you were a health risk (to charge more money for their insurance).

They got updated in '83 and have since become full of color and funky graphics. Despite these changes, the basic idea is wrong. The length of your bones (your height) and the force you exert on *Earth* (your weight), don't explain everything.

Even people of the same height or weight (or both), can vary massively in other ways. Some may carry more muscle, some might have short legs or long collar bones, and all these sorts of factors are things that charts can't see. They're blind to reality.

The point on the chart where height and weight meet, is a point compared to another *Jane's* points, i.e. they're averages. Averages are simply what's common. And when it comes to health, *common* does not mean *ideal*. Think about it.

Today's charts divide everyone into neat little groups. Underweight, normal, overweight, obese, and the scary sounding, *morbidly obese*. They're just words! They simply make it easier for others to describe you.

Height and weight charts used to *only* be found in insurance company offices. Gradually they made their way into doctor's surgeries, then gyms, and now they're available everywhere. When you see one, don't bother looking. You know better.

BODY MASS INDEX

It's amazing, you just need to take three normal words, stick them together, and it all sounds so scientific! Body - Mass - Index, or BMI for short. This is where you or your doctor gets out a calculator.

BMI uses mathematics to work out how much mass you have compared to your height. Take your height in inches and multiply itself. Then divide your weight in pounds by that answer. Are you confused or bored? I'm both!

Just like the height and weight tables, there are charts which work out your BMI. As with all charts, this doesn't make the figures any more useful. BMI also likes to divide itself into neat little groups.

Their categories sound like a mixture of the classics, underweight, normal, overweight, and types of space ship, Obese Class I, Obese Class II and Obese Class III. You can see why they never became high school insults!

I now suggest that you forget all those categories, forever. What's strange, is that we *had* forgotten them for years, over 150 in fact. BMI was actually invented in the 1830s by a Belgian mathematician. He sounded fun!

When people started to question the accuracy of height and weight tables, BMI made a comeback. It may sound complicated, but it's not different than what we've seen before. And like height and weight tables, BMI is everywhere.

The formula only works in the extremely under or overweight, although by that point, it's kind of obvious! Annoyingly, in the commonest BMI group of *normal*, there's the smallest amount of accuracy. Doh!

The reason its accuracy is so poor, is back to an old friend, *Average Jane*. BMI figures came from studying all the data from lots of *Janes*. By now you can see that if *Jane* wasn't ideal, and we measured lots of *Janes*, we could be very lost!

It's time to add three letters, and say goodbye: RIP – BMI. It's too mechanical, and not personal enough to tell you anything worthwhile. So, we've ditched tables and statistics, and now you're still thinking, 'just tell me how fat I am'!

BODY FAT PERCENTAGE

I promise, it's the last method to ignore! In the quest for more knowledge about our bodies, science has apparently delivered the ultimate statistic, your percent body fat. Sometimes it's called your body composition.

Now out of all the measures we've discussed, your percentage of body fat deserves credit for trying. I'll give it an A+ for effort. Knowing how much of your body is fat and how much isn't, is a logical place to start.

To find this figure out, you can either pinch yourself (with giant plastic tweezers), get dunked under water, have your breathing analyzed, let electricity pass through you, or even get scanned by a huge X-ray type machine.

These methods vary in their accuracy. They all give you a number explaining how much of you is made from fat. The left-over percentage is the combined total of your water, muscle, organs and bone.

Let's assume that you got your body fat percentage measured accurately. The results are in, and now what? Time for another table, chart or opinion! Oh yes, they'll always find a way back to haunt you!

All these are also made up by analyzing results from more people. Depending on where you look, you will find different meanings for your body fat percentage tests. There's a big problem. These meanings are meaningless!

Scientific research can tell you lots about body fat levels. Olympic male athletes are less than 10% fat, women with 15% or less stop having periods, and if you get below 3%, you'll probably never get out of bed again.

Surprisingly, even body fat percentage has problems. Say you have two people with 20% fat. They could even be the same height. One might still have a big tummy or thighs, and the other might appear to have a balanced body.

This happens because of differences in muscle and fat cell location, bone length and water content. Your body fat percentage is like knowing the ingredient list for a cake recipe. It can't tell you how the cake will turn out.

The problem with body fat percentage is the same as all the other methods we've looked at. They're rarely accurate, they

18

only compare you to others, and they create numbers which just scare you or give you false hope.

From a purely visual point of view, they're almost laughable. When was the last time you walked down the street, saw someone who impressed or shocked you, and thought, 'wow, they must have a BMI of 19' or be 'obese class III'!

So, I think by now you realize that modern measuring techniques can be fun at most, but definitely a distraction from what we all go back to in the end: how we see ourselves, how we see others, and how we compare what we see.

The scientists who just read that are now pulling their hair out in rage. They prefer to live in a world of exact data, research and theory. That's really not a world that most of us live in. I've got a theory. **We don't do theory!**

So, what's left? Oh, that big question, 'how fat do you think I am?'. Can you see the answer yet? I just gave you a big hint. The answer has the same number of letters as fat. No? It's about what you *see*.

Don't tear up the page or throw your phone! I'm simply recommending that you rely on the most powerful, personal and instinctive method of judgment available. Your brain. You're probably shaking it right now!

The purpose of this section is to hit home how important it is to **trust yourself**, *and* to **compare yourself to yourself**. Okay, I can't stop you making comparisons with your friends. And besides, just read the subtitle of the book!

But it's crucial that you develop trust in what's physical, i.e. real. Doing this will encourage self-honesty. Once you get that and stop relying on others, you'll know exactly when it's right for you to carry on as normal, or to push harder.

Some of you may have a habit of relying on what others believe, either by asking friends, family or even online strangers what they think of your body. I hereby give you official permission to stop that! Right now! I said NOW!

And by the way, I'm not suggesting that you never weigh yourself again. Used right, weighing scales are still a reliable and motivational tool. There are other things that you can use, and I'm sure that some of you already do.

THE MIRROR

Looking in this is probably the closest thing you can get to an honest opinion from an outsider! If you use one, make sure it's neutral (doesn't make you look skinnier or fatter than you really are). And of course, always use the same one.

If you really want to get a good opinion of your body, don't just look at your front or side view. **Get another mirror to see what's behind you**. This isn't encouraging you to become obsessed. It's simply inaccurate to ignore half your image!

If you can't do that, visit a clothing store's changing room. The lighting's often nasty, but it allows you to get detailed info on your body's overall look. Keep visiting the same store. And no, you don't have to buy anything!

CLOTHES

This isn't as simple as it sounds. There's probably nothing better than being able to fit snuggly into your favorite pair of jeans, especially if you've been struggling for a while. If you're using one pair for this comparison, it's a great tool.

Unfortunately, those sneaky numbers have made their way back into town: clothing sizes. They can be very misleading. Fashion designers realize that we all like to fit the smallest size possible.

Because of this, some will size their clothes large. Imagine you're facing a close call between two similar but different brands of jeans. One's a size 8 and the other is a 6. Wouldn't you be tempted to buy the feel-good size 6?

You can also make it more difficult for yourself by using an item of clothing that *changes* size. Natural fabrics like cotton can shrink dramatically, especially if you dry them artificially. Some items can also dramatically loosen too!

So, to use clothes as a guide, keep some items aside that stay constant. And don't panic if you fit easily in one store's jeans, but really struggle into some from another. No one gains weight that quickly! It's just numbers.

PHOTOS

Digital photography using a phone or camera makes keeping track of your progress easy. You don't even require anyone's help. Just a clever place to position a camera or tripod. Photos in front of a full-length mirror work well too.

To use photos, you need to be consistent. That means taking them from the same spot, having the same lighting (important) and using the same camera. If you're wearing a swimsuit or shorts, keep those the same too.

So, you're going to rely on yourself, the mirror, your clothes, and maybe take some photos. As I mentioned before, weighing scales are useful too. They get their own section. But for now, I can hear you shouting another question!

HOW MUCH DO YOU THINK I CAN LOSE?

For some, this might be the second most important question you want answered. And in fact, it's the *easiest* one to answer. But it will also be the most difficult truth to accept from the whole book. Are you ready? Take a deep breath.

There's no limit on how much fat you can lose. If you're very fat, you can lose a bigger total compared to those who have less fat to start with. But everyone, and that means e-v-e-r-y-o-n-e, can be skinny. Yes, skinny.

Scientists and psychologists probably find that irresponsible. I don't care. I just want you to find it inspiring. If it's making you angry, I understand. We've all overheard conversations and absorbed stuff that suggests being skinny isn't for everyone.

'You really must realize that you're not made like her'

'I guess I just have a super fast metabolism'

'Genes are the most important thing'

'Come on, look at your ankles'

If you hear something enough, you'll start to believe it, make it a fact, and finally you'll live up to it. It's wrong that so many people do this and give up their dream of being skinny. It's time to wipe the hard drive!

Being skinny is for everyone. It's healthy, it's possible, and importantly, it's how the human body loves to be.

While scientists and diet gurus have been studying the *differences* between human beings, they've forgotten to spend more time looking at *similarities*. And as it turns out, there's quite a lot.

We already have enough knowledge, which if properly understood and used, can keep us skinny and healthy. This will work for at least 99% of the population. Even those in the other 1% can improve beyond their dreams.

You might be wondering how this can be true, especially as skinny success seems quite rare. Human beings are part of the universe. And that's full of laws. The laws of physics, chemistry and biology are three well-known ones.

You have never 'failed' on any diet. Never! The diet has failed to be properly designed and apply these basic laws.

Big difference. You've got to delete any sense of failu...Or you'll believe that you're special in the wrong way and be 'one of those' who can't be skinny. Don't become another amateur expert on genetics, i.e. don't blame your genes!

HOW QUICKLY DO YOU THINK I COULD LOSE IT?

No one can deny that some people lose fat quicker than others, and with less effort. This difference in speed causes people to give up. The crucial thing to realize is that eventually, you can look as skinny as you like.

I sense that was too wishy washy an answer for you! Of all the questions, it's the speed issue that excites most. Maybe it's *the* reason you chose *Six Weeks To OMG*. I'm going to give you the best, honest answer I can.

In a way, I could have answered this via the previous question, 'how much do you think I could lose?'. But it needed a time frame to be more accurate. **In 6 weeks, you can lose between 10 and 20 pounds of fat**. Not *weight*.

That means, if you apply the ideas of the book, you will **lose fat at the rate of up to 3.5 pounds every week**. If this disappoints you, hold up. Many diets promise faster weight loss. And they do. But it's weight, not fat.

Many people, assume that fast weight loss is water loss. Nope. When calories are slashed ultra low (or food choices become really limited), most of the weight is muscle loss. And that's a natural disaster!

Water loss is *easy* to fix. The body has built-in mechanisms to keep you interested in water or watery foods. Even if you keep ignoring your thirst, your body will make you think again by slowing you down and making you physically weak.

In fact, room temperature water can go from mouth to muscles in under 10 minutes. But muscles themselves takes weeks, months and sometimes even *years* to rebuild and recover from a sudden loss. And during that time, you will suffer.

Some of you might be thinking, 'so what, no one can see it, and anyway I look skinny!'. Shrinking your muscles isn't really a yay moment. You can hide it from others, but your body always knows what's going on.

Losing muscle is never a good idea. In a cosmetic sense, you'll have a slightly softer body. Maybe you can deal with that. Next up, is the development of a reduced metabolism. Finally, something to blame being fat on!

Muscle is where most of our food is 'burned'. Think of muscle as an oven. Shrink your oven, and you shrink your ability to burn calories. And a smaller oven equals less slices of pizza for you!

So, back to those 10 to 20 pounds. That works out to be a weekly fat loss rate of roughly 1.5 to 3.5 pounds. Can you lose it faster? Yes. I've seen faster fat loss in about 10% of people. And, I've seen slower.

What causes this variation? The truthful answer is that I don't know. There are so many factors at play, many of which we haven't discovered yet. And because we don't know what we're looking for, I can't suggest how to improve them.

10 to 20 pounds of fat loss in 6 weeks is fast. It happens when you get lots of things right. If up to 3.5 pounds per week sounds slow, think how losing that week after week soon adds up. I bet you didn't even gain that fast!

When people lose more weight than this, they usually don't look better. When you get 10 to 20 pounds of fat loss in 6 weeks (even if you're 250 to start), the changes you have made will be obvious to anyone. As in, 'OMG' obvious!

Your clothes will fit better, with especially good slimming around your waist (where fat can sit deep inside you). Your face, neck and jawline will be less puffy. And you'll feel lighter, a feeling that's *so* refreshing.

Okay, take a few moments to think about what you've read in this section. It's probably been thought changing, confusing and even tiring. Be honest with yourself, and move to the next section when you're ready. That's decision time!

GET THE SKINNY ON...

OMG 6 Everyone has an opinion but yours is always best

OMG 5 Forget about tables, charts, percentages or BMI

OMG 4 Weighing scales, the mirror and clothes are good motivators

OMG 3 You can lose between 10 and 20 pounds of fat in 6 weeks

OMG 2 Going faster could mean losing too much muscle (bad)

OMG 1 Everyone can get super skinny despite what others say

OMG ! Start to trust in yourself and you'll be rewarded!

BIG PLANS

We all have different goals, so we need different plans. Choosing the right one is simple, just be honest. And by that, I mean be accurate about how much and how fast you need to lose fat. I'm not asking you to be easy on yourself either!

I realize that for some, even 6 weeks is just too long. Maybe you've got a big party coming up, or it's holidays, or you just want to hurry. If your target is 15 pounds or less, you could choose the hardest plan, and lose it sooner than 6 weeks.

There is a limit to this high-speed approach though, and certain amounts of fat loss are not likely, no matter what other books, trainers or gurus say. The truth is, most diets or health programs simply pick numbers out of thin air.

You're better than that. The amounts I've targeted are not based on guess work. They're from experiments. And I mean, experiments *officially tested on humans!* They're pretty much the average upper limit for fat loss in 6 weeks.

Like all averages, some people will lose less, and some people will lose more. Stop it! 'Stop what?', you're thinking. Well, at this point many people lose confidence. They decide that they'll be the one person who loses less. Repeat after me:

I don't know who I really am, until I've really tried!

27

I don't know who I really am, until I've really tried!

I don't know who I really am, until I've really tried!

If you're struggling, you might want to shift down a level, and go back up when you can. Try not to mix and match all the time, as this could get you into a habit of wishy washy discipline.

To be clear, the basic ideas of the book are very similar for all of you. Only in a few areas are there differences, and this is where you'll see a variation written. If there's no mention of a plan variation, it means do it all! Think of video game levels:

WAVE

LOSE 10 POUNDS OF FAT IN 6 WEEKS

This is the easiest level. Being the easiest doesn't mean it's easy! Many ideas in this book will be new and controversial, and if you're worried about adjusting your brain and lifestyle to the shock, this could be the one for you.

On *Wave*, you'll be waking up your body and mind to a new way of working. If 10 pounds of fat loss happens to be your target, but you want to lose it quicker than 6 weeks, you could try the next level of intensity, *Blaze*.

BLAZE

LOSE 15 POUNDS OF FAT IN 6 WEEKS

This plan is tougher than *Wave*. It needs more discipline and mental strength from you. But by using more movement, plus smarter food choices with better biochemistry and physics, *Blaze* will generate about 50% more fat burning than *Wave*.

If you really want to go for the maximum amount of fat loss in 6 weeks, or lose less but do it at warp speed, then you could try the final level, *Quake*. It's not easy, but in return, your body will simply have to start looking exactly as you want.

QUAKE

LOSE 20 POUNDS OF FAT IN 6 WEEKS

Make no mistake, this level requires a real shift in beliefs and effort compared to most things you may have tried before. Your friends will think you're crazy, and you might say to yourself at times, 'what am I doing?'!

But the results will speak for themselves. *Quake* requires even smarter choices than *Blaze*, and even more dedication. If you're still not sure, sit down, re-read the previous chapter, sleep on it, and decide in the morning.

To repeat, though there are 3 levels, the principles stay the same. To lose more, some things obviously need to be tougher. Think of *Wave*, *Blaze* and *Quake* as *easy*, *normal* and *hard*. Or hard, harder and 'are you serious?'. I'm joking. Not!

SOME NOTES FOR NON-BELIEVERS

Critics could suggest that these plans aren't practical for constant use. And you know what, if you were to feel like you were constantly on a plan, any plan, they'd be right. But they're not right about everything. Critics never are!

I *want* you to feel like you're on a plan *in the beginning*, as this will excite and energize you. But after a while, you'll start to understand how stuff works, and these techniques will gradually melt their way into your life. Plan? What plan!

Carrying extra fat is massively unhealthy, linked to lots of diseases, makes you feel miserable, and only happens because of extra-ordinary behaviors. To fight back, **we need an extra-ordinary plan**.

What about those who say that the fat loss targets are too low? Perhaps you agree with them. There's no such thing as too little fat loss. Yes, we all want things faster, but **every ounce of fat that you lose is progress in the right direction**.

Experts who claim that you can lose fat faster than 20 pounds in 6 weeks are not experts. They're just random number generators! But maybe you remember a time when someone you knew lost more. Maybe it was you. Here's how it happens.

SUCCESS BY WEIGHT ONLY

This often means losing more than fat. As I mentioned before, assuming 'it's just water weight' is wrong. Losing extreme amounts of weight quickly means losing extreme amounts of muscle. You've got to love your muscles! Why?

They contain our big well of water, they get us out of bed, look after our immune system, and they use up the energy in that sneaky *second* bar of chocolate! For those just interested in appearance, losing muscle will make you squishy to touch.

In the past few years, many diets have caused massive weight loss. Their inventors have claimed that some of this is water, and that it can be made safe by *just drinking more*. This is either stupidity or lies. **Massive weight loss always involves losing muscle**.

EXCESSIVE EXERCISE

Being physical is great. In fact, it's how we're meant to be. But even cavemen would have rested from time to time. Why? Because our ancestors had real experience of experiencing exhaustion.

Muscle cells develop very small tears when used. This is completely normal, and up to a point, our body can easily fix them. Go beyond this, and it starts to go wrong. And it's not just muscles that suffer if you over-exercise.

First to go is your immunity, so you get coughs and colds. Next to go are your joints. You could find yourself twisting an ankle too often, or even tearing an entire muscle, tendon or ligament. Trust me, sitting injured makes it easy to get fat!

Eventually, the body's chemical system has problems. Men lose testosterone, and women lose estrogen. Apart from making guys more like girls, and girls more like guys, this all leads to the final problem. Feeling sad.

Physical activity is great for the mind, but when you rely on it too much, the body simply can't recover and does anything to stop you hurting it. And what's the easiest way for it to do this? It depresses you! That's exactly what nature does.

How much is too much? For most people, doing more than 2 hours per day will cause problems. Our plans use physical activity, but it's more about **timing and combining** it with other principles, instead of just doing lots.

CONSTANTLY BAD FOOD CHOICES

If a diet tells you to live on a limited number of foods, you're in trouble from the start. I don't care how good it is, no human can *just* live on chocolate! Diet recipes may look interesting, but subconsciously they limit you.

Many diets are designed knowing that we understand the dangers of being fat. And with that, they have the perfect excuse to persuade you to live on just a few foods. **Skinnier is healthier, but you must get the basics right**.

Nature doesn't want us to get serious disease, so it gives us nutrients to prevent it. Trouble is, it scatters them in a wide variety of foods. Eat just a few, and you might not get enough of the magical mix to protect you.

SUPER COMPLICATED DESIGN

Many diets are designed by those who realize, if something doesn't look complicated, people won't believe it. It's crazy, but many of us have a natural habit of assuming that simple things can't be useful. You know, 'it can't be *that* easy'.

So, diets got complicated. Your body isn't impressed by complication *or* simplicity. It just knows what works, and what doesn't.

Many diets are so complicated that they never let you forget that you're on one!

This book may appear complex to start with. But once you understand it, everything will become very simple. And if you've been on a diet before, this new knowledge will help you spot the reasons why they *didn't* work.

DRUGS

Okay, here's the truth. There are drugs that speed up weight loss, fat loss, or any kind of loss you want. Some are street drugs, some are medical, but what they all have in common, is that eventually, they *will* stop working.

Either that, or they'll stop *you* working. Governments in a panic have tried to use many of these drugs to reduce the levels of obesity, but even they know that it's a shortcut that often goes wrong. All drugs have some kind of side-effect.

Some side-effects can't be lived with, and others can. In fact, I'll encourage you to use a drug later. But it's not one that's smuggled into the country. You can buy it from a grocery store, it's safe, and it helps.

HARDLY EATING OR CHUCKING IT UP

Time to talk about the elephant in the room. The 'A' word and the 'B' word. **Anorexia**, hardly eating, and **Bulimia**, eating but vomiting. They're more common than we realize or admit. Many parents and friends actually turn a blind eye.

33

They're common because of a dangerous triple whammy. One, our desire to look good. Two, a lack of decent diet info. And three, the big one, deep emotional issues which drive people to use food as something other than fuel or fun.

What's that? **In most people with eating disorders, food becomes an alter ego**. It becomes a version of themselves which can be *controlled*. We all hate chaos, and if we can't control our thoughts, we *will* control something.

I'm not here to cure Anorexia and Bulimia. Even the idea of a cure is ridiculous. Sufferers need support, understanding, and time. It takes time to see ourselves properly, and this can't be made to fast forward.

I'm talking about Anorexia and Bulimia in terms of those relatively rare people who do it purely to look better. If you starve yourself, eventually, you will become very, very thin. And very, very ill.

However active you are, your brain is always working. It demands up to a quarter of your calories. Plus your heart keeps ticking, organs keep doing their jobs, and you always lose a bit of heat. Even couch potatoes burn calories.

Anorexia sufferers know with certainty, that eating less makes their body skinny. The problem is, we're not only designed to become *Victoria's Secret* models. We're designed to win *Weakest Link* and *Wipeout* too.

We're made to be brilliant at lots of things, and that requires lots of nutrients. Not so much that you create an excess (fat), but enough to build the most complex design on the planet. Over the long-term, our nutrient list *must* be brilliant.

Your body is only 8 years old. Yes, I mean yours! If you looked at any of the cells in your body, and checked how old they are, they'd be a maximum of about 8 years old. This is because we're constantly being worn out, and then, re-made.

Cells in your stomach might be replaced every 3 hours. New cells in your skin start every 3 weeks. Parts of your teeth are just 2 years old. In simple terms, we are constantly rolling along a kind of factory conveyor belt.

This means, we literally are what we eat. We're all 'asked' by the human body to go to the grocery store, and buy the nutrients it needs. Anorexia sufferers refuse to buy anything on this list, or only buy some of the items.

If that list was supposed to be for a cake, you just wouldn't be able to bake a good one. And that's what happens with the massive weight loss in Anorexia sufferers. They shrink down, but what they're made of, is junk.

Eat poorly for 3 weeks, and cells who are born at the bottom layer of your skin will surface looking like they've slept in the *Grand Canyon*. These underfed critters will show up as weak, stretch-mark prone, dull looking skin.

Keep eating badly, and you'll start affecting the cells which take longer to grow. Organs, brain and eventually your teeth. Tip to toe. *Including* your toes. **Being skinny by not eating much always leads to a problem in the end**.

With Bulimia, it's slightly different. Some are part-time Anorexia sufferers too, going through long periods of hardly eating at all. This means getting most of the problems we've just discussed. But they get new problems too.

When you've got Bulimia, you might look skinny without looking ill, and hold your weight down with no one getting suspicious. A good actress can appear completely normal in public, apart from the frequent bathroom visits.

Vomiting literally reverses calorie intake. And therefore, it causes dramatic weight loss, at least temporarily. Nature always catches up. Vomit is extremely acidic, easily destroying teeth, but also the throat (making it more vulnerable to cancer).

With careful use of breath mints and lots of water to clear the acid, some of this stuff can be hidden. However, it's absolutely impossible to hide certain things from the body. And I mean, impossible.

Gradually, various big organs like skin and stomach will suffer and start to go wrong. But much more slowly, and in ways we still don't understand, **appetite centers** screw up. Appetite centers?

Noticing food, enjoying it, craving it and knowing when to ignore it, all get decided by parts of the brain. These areas are complex, and they're linked in to your general feelings of happiness. That's appetite centers.

Training them with certain principles (like this book) is a good idea, because modern life has thrown them off track. But by eating food and vomiting it up, you cause massive confusion to the brain.

You're re-wiring extremely complex areas, and even the human super computer doesn't have an emergency plan. Bulimia sufferers develop a long-term strange relationship to food, one that even they can't explain.

Anorexia and Bulimia will make you lose weight. There's no denying it. But the weight loss itself is never usually a problem, other than what members of the public, family or friends find visually acceptable.

The problem is making the body from a limited grocery list of ingredients, and also re-wiring our amazing neck-top computer, the brain. If you do this for 2 years or more, you're in serious trouble. Find some help. It *will* be okay.

Humans are blessed with a miracle-like ability to get better. Because of the unique way we're built, cell by cell, we get the chance to start fresh, from the minute we make a decision to do so.

THE NEW BABY ELEPHANT

For most people, Anorexia and Bulimia are still very private problems. Not for celebrities though. The constant growth of digital media, especially the internet, has changed their lives forever. And like all humans, celebs have problems too.

Many high-profile cases, particularly including actresses and female musicians, have raised the profile of eating disorders to staggering new heights. Shocking pictures with gory details have been beamed into our homes and onto our phones.

This exposure, combined with the general rise of information has given birth to a new baby elephant. It's called **Orthorexia**. It's a made-up word, roughly from the Greek, *correct* and *appetite*. And the number of sufferers is huge.

What is a sufferer though? **An orthorexic is someone with an unhealthy obsession with food**. Some might say that reading this book makes *you* one. And I would agree if I'd written the book in a certain style. But I didn't.

This book gives you facts, and hopefully, in a user-friendly way. I aim to encourage understanding, not obsession. I've found that once you get to the truth of a subject, any obsession tends to dampen down immediately.

I also believe that if you're reading this, you have an obsession with your body, not food itself. It's just that the two are closely linked. A *temporary* obsession with your body and food *is* healthy, especially if it draws you closer to the calming truth.

Back to the orthorexics. They used to be a tiny hardcore bunch that chose to hang around health stores instead of malls. But because information is only a *Wiki* away, they've dragged their behaviors into general grocery stores.

In some ways, the rise of Orthorexia has brought about many positive changes in our food supply. Companies know that we're generally a smart bunch now, and this has pressured them to produce cleaner, organic and generally more wholesome products.

But there's a downside to being an Orthorexic. It means seeing food purely as a *noun*. A thing. Fuel. Something to measure, control and use. And that's a shame, because food is so much more than that.

Food is a *feeling*, and eating it is almost a ritual. Okay, eating at a drive-thru is hardly that! Actually, I'm not sure, because even that can become a pleasurable occasion. That's it, thank you brain. Food is often *an occasion*. And life *needs* a sense of occasion.

There have been some calls for Orthorexia to be classified as an eating disorder. I don't think it's that. And I don't believe that Anorexia or Bulimia are eating disorders either. They're mind problems. Food just happens to tag along.

Anorexia, Bulimia and Orthorexia are the physical result of non-physical problems. If you think you have any of them, you need a check-up from the neck up. Alternatively, reach into your heart. It's full of answers and honesty. Feel it. *Connect.*

If you're Orthorexic, you might not feel alone as some Anorexics or Bulimics. In some ways, that makes your situation worse. But any long-term obsession isn't good, because it takes up valuable space in your brain.

Space that would be much better off thinking about random stuff, fun stuff and stuff I can't even think up a name for. I urge you to become an expert as quickly as possible, and yet don't seek perfection of knowledge. It never arrives.

This book will give you a nice chunk of smarts to get you feeling ahead of the pack. But truly, don't dwell on diet or just looks, including the looks of others. There's so much more to life. **Fly out of your cage today**.

TAKE YOUR PICK

There are two purposes for this section. Firstly, to introduce you to the plans and let you choose how much you want to lose. Secondly, to show you that going faster is risky. I am not criticizing any particular diet. Just all which disagree!

Losing fat quickly is exciting. And so is keeping it off. To do this, you need a body and brain that works normally. If anything encourages you to skip over that, think about the long-term honestly, and be smart. **Always be long-term smart**.

Right, to make choosing a plan simple, instead of using complicated tables or diagrams, I've written the options as sentences. Read them aloud, see what sounds right. And then we can move forwards.

In 6 weeks, I want to lose 10 pounds. I'll do **WAVE**.

In 6 weeks, I want to lose 15 pounds. I'll do **BLAZE**.

In 6 weeks, I want to lose 20 pounds. I'll do **QUAKE**.

In 4 weeks, I want to lose 10 pounds. I'll do **BLAZE**.

In 4 weeks, I want to lose 15 pounds. I'll do **QUAKE**.

In 3 weeks, I want to lose 10 pounds. I'll do **QUAKE**.

If you need to lose more than 20 pounds or less than 10, the most important thing is to **make a start**. Pick one. However much you need to lose, at some point, you might want to re-adjust your goals and change levels.

GET THE SKINNY ON...

OMG 6 Pick a plan based on your gut feeling

OMG 5 Losing 15 lbs or less can be done faster than 6 weeks

OMG 4 Your body is built cell by cell with a complex grocery list

OMG 3 Super fast weight loss results in general health problems

OMG 2 Eating disorders are the physical results of mind problems

OMG 1 Avoid any thing or person that risks your long-term happiness

OMG ! Pick a plan and go for it baby!

MEASURING GREATNESS

As you read this, millions of people around the world will be getting on and off weighing scales. Some will be leaning to one side, a few will be naked, and most will be holding their b-b-b-b-breath!

Everyone likes to measure their success. It's natural. Apart from the numbers in our bank balance, it seems that the numbers on weighing scales make a difference to our happiness. With so much resting on it, you might as well do it properly.

BUY YOUR OWN

If you can't afford some, save up quick. Scales are great when they're accurate, and *pointless* when they're not. The easiest way to reduce their accuracy, is to overuse them. And the easiest way to overuse them, is for many people to use them.

If you're used to weighing yourself at a gym, stop right now! These scales maybe used 100 times per day, or more. That's like you using them twice a week for a year, in *one* day! Even commercial scales can't take that.

If gym scales say you've lost lots of weight, you'll feel great. But what if they're inaccurate? If they say you've gained *tons*, then how do you feel? **When it comes to your feelings, you need accuracy**. Buy some scales. But which kind?

GO DIGITAL

Some scales have circular plastic dials, and some have electronic displays. Although scales with dials can be highly accurate, the advantage of digital scales is that changes in weight can be clearly displayed in small amounts.

This is useful, because **over a day, fat loss happens in small chunks**. These constant little improvements can be exciting and boost confidence. The best scales show differences as small as 2 ounces in the US, or 50 grams in Europe.

Buy some from a well-known company, one with a reputation to lose if their product was poor. And forget about fancy features. BMI, body fat and *spoken* weight are all gimmicks! You just need accuracy.

GET OFF THE RED CARPET!

Manufacturers always include instructions that suggest scales need a hard floor to work properly. Guess what? No one reads instructions! Instead of not selling you scales, they've developed scales with carpet feet. No, no, no!

Carpets get tread on all day. They change. All the special carpet feet in the world can't stop scales from wobbling! So, to get wobble-free accuracy, find the most solid floor you can, and always stick to the same spot. Stand on a road if you have to!

WHEN SHALL I WEIGH MYSELF?

Simple. In the morning, and ideally, after you've *been* to the bathroom! That way, you'll have reliable accuracy. The time on the clock doesn't matter. It's just important to not let random water weight affect your perception of success. So make sure that you *go* first!

Throughout the day, our eating and drinking patterns make a huge difference. Any excitement through changes in fluid levels is a false victory. Water levels go up and down for endless reasons, but they rarely change how we look.

When we eat carbohydrates, some are stored *inside* our muscles. The level of this can increase dramatically from morning to night. Each bit of carbs we store inside our muscles drags in 2.4 times that amount of water.

You could easily have low stores of carbs in your muscles in the morning, and throughout the day, increase them by around 14 oz. (400 grams). In addition to your weight changing by this amount, you'll also be sucking in water.

This means that just through regular eating and drinking, you could appear to weigh 2 pounds (1 kilo) heavier in the evening, without changing your actual body fat at all! **Be consistent and measure in the mornings only**.

HOW OFTEN SHALL I WEIGH MYSELF?

Not every day! That's the quick answer. We've just seen how much weight changes from morning to night. **I would suggest**

weighing yourself no more than once per week. Once every two weeks is better, but no one can handle it!

7 days is enough time for you to burn some serious energy. In combination with scales that display small changes in weight, that's perfect. Go for *Monday mornings* and get the figures that will inspire you to work hard the whole week.

GET NAKED

The most consistent item of clothing you own, is your skin. If I had a dollar for every time someone was heavy on the scales and said, 'it's my jeans', I'd have a lot of dollars! Close your door, get naked, and get accurate. You'll avoid criticism too.

GET THE SKINNY ON...

OMG 6 Measuring weight is still a useful motivator

OMG 5 Use scales which can show small improvements

OMG 4 Use them on a solid floor and never carpet

OMG 3 Measure in the morning to avoid carb weight confusion

OMG 2 Weigh yourself once per week at most

OMG 1 Get on the scales naked for maximum consistency

OMG ! Buy your own scales and keep them hidden!

BREAK FAST OR BREAK FATS

'Don't skip breakfast'

'Never skip breakfast'

'People who don't eat breakfast get fat'

'Breakfast is the most important meal of the day'

'You've got to break your fast'

'A good breakfast sets you up for the whole day'

'If you eat breakfast, you won't need to pig out later'

'Eat this special breakfast and you'll lose weight'

'You just can't function without breakfast'

'She's so unhealthy, she hardly ever eats breakfast'

'Breakfast helps you concentrate'

'Eat your breakfast, now!'

That's a dozen breakfast rules for you. Ever heard some of them? Maybe all twelve? THEY'RE NOT TRUE! This section is probably the most important one you'll read. Nonsense rules are there to be broken, even if it's scary.

Starting tomorrow, or whenever you begin your plan, I want you to stop eating breakfast. Yes, *skip* breakfast! You might need to hide it or give to a homeless person (or a non-overweight hungry hound). Curious yet? Great, keep reading!

Understand what follows, and you'll be a long way towards being permanently skinny. Cereal manufacturers would love to burn what I'm saying, your brain might find it hard to believe, and at first, your stomach will wish you hadn't read it.

Give it a chance. Once you really get it, and once your body really gets it, it will be much easier to stick to every day. It's a chunky chapter that will help you be less chunky! So, why do we eat breakfast?

BREAKFAST TASTES NICE

But why does it seem to taste *so* nice? Well, although you've been asleep for hours, your brain has actually been up all night, keeping the body going, and organizing repairs. This night shift takes **energy**.

When you go to bed, there's a small amount of energy left in your system. There could be food in your tummy from your last meal, some in your blood, and a bit stored away in your liver. Scientists call saved energy in the liver, **glycogen**.

One of our liver's main functions is to give us boosts of energy when we haven't eaten for a while. It's like an emergency back-pack inside us. It takes glycogen, a fancy word for **stored carbs**, and trickles it out for the night shift workers.

By the time you wake up, there's no energy left in the system. Everything in your tummy is gone (so *that's* why it's so flat in the morning!), everything in your blood is gone, and your liver is pretty much out of gas too.

The brain senses that you're running low, so it makes you hungry. It makes your tummy r-u-m-b-l-e! It's freaking out, literally not knowing where your next meal is coming from. So, it sends you out into the wilderness (kitchen) to find it.

BECAUSE IT'S THERE

Our body's genetics are old. They came from a time when food wasn't guaranteed. Cavemen couldn't instantly milk a cow, toast up some waffles or call for pizza! **Our genes are from a time when getting food was like winning the lottery**.

After 2,000,000 birthdays, our human body has held up well. Okay, we stopped using our appendix and speak smoother, but we're generally *the same*. Unlike the world. That's changed *lots*. The body doesn't know this. We live in times of plenty.

This is more true if you have spare body fat to lose, a source of energy that's as plentiful as your own shopping cart full of breakfast food. If getting fed was still a lottery, modern humans would be jackpot winners every day!

IT'S BIG BUSINESS

Next time you go to a food store, take a closer look at the cereal lane. It will take up lots of space, be neatly stacked full of color, and it will have so much variety, that if you can't find something you like the look of, you'll feel fussy!

This area of a food store makes the most profit. The products are cheap to make, with most of a cereal company's cash being spent on pricey advertising. Or paying celebrities who don't eat the stuff, to say that they do!

They know that if they find a taste or an idea that you like first thing in the morning, you'll be a hooked customer for a very long time. How many other foods types do that? The easiest way to addict you is to add sugar. Brains lap it up.

Cereals crops only entered our diet 10,000 years ago. For a few million years before, we got on fine without them. What did we eat? Definitely *not* cereal. In fact, we couldn't and wouldn't have eaten anything first thing after waking up.

So that's breakfast. It tastes good because our bodies are virtually empty in the morning, it's freely available, and big business keeps selling us the stuff. This all adds up to millions of breakfast lovers every morning.

'GOTTA HAVE MY BOWL, GOTTA HAVE CEREAL'

Rebecca Black sung those lyrics over 200,000,000 times on *YouTube*. And of course, everyone eats breakfast. So, are they right? NO! **Popularity isn't always for a good reason**. And the first reason *why* we eat breakfast, is actually the biggest reason to avoid it.

Move the body when it has little energy floating around it, and energy will have to come from somewhere. Your body fat.

Why? It's simple. Imagine you're a car, and you need gas (calories) to drive (live). Where would you get it from? Well hello, what about the gas tank? This is the fastest place for the car to get gas from.

Push the pedal (e.g. move, think, sing!), and you've got gas. In the body, the gas tank is like our blood, our liver, and the inside of our muscles. They contain all the energy from the food or drink you've been having.

Throughout the day, we 'cars' stop by gas stations to fill up. We eat! Whenever you do this, you're topping up the energy in the tank (blood, liver, muscles). And when there's energy in the tank, why would the body use anything else?

But remember that in the morning, you've had the engine on all night. That being your brain and other organs. Those cheeky nippers have been sipping at your gas in the dark! And actually, that's *great*. You wake up with almost no gas.

With no gas in the tank, the body is pushed to do something radical. If you insist on going out for a drive (i.e. move!), it lets you do so, and it powers you by burning your body fat. No gas in the tank, means no other choice.

When you first skip breakfast, it's difficult. You've had years of being used to the easy life of *instant* food. And that's made your body adapt. Given time, it will adapt back. **You will get better at burning your body fat**.

During this time, you'll get some loud tummy rumbling! This is also due to changes in the rest of your diet. And, you might find it harder to concentrate. Again, give your body time, and it will adapt to focus with ease.

But immediately, your body will start burning much more fat. **Only after a long sleep does this happen**. This rare window of opportunity *must* be used. If you don't, think of it as wasting 8 hours of preparation time (sleeping)!

Some experts, and just as many cereal manufacturers, claim that skipping breakfast makes you eat more in total. That can be true in the short term. But even then, this just hides the most important fact.

And that fact, which they can't deny or dare mention, is that **eating food first thing in the morning stops all fat burning**. *Instantly.* When food has just entered the body, there is no reason for the body to start burning stored calories. Why bother!

If you ask a crowd of diet experts to raise their hands if they believe skipping breakfast is wrong, every hand will go up. So what? You can't find the truth by simply counting hands. They're wrong and I'm right. **Our genes are right**. If you want to lose body fat fast, be bold. **Skip breakfast**.

At some point in their lives, most people have skipped a breakfast. Maybe it was deliberate, or maybe it was due to being in a hurry. And when they did it, they felt awful. They therefore came to the conclusion, I *should* eat breakfast.

But that situation only happens because we are *so* used to having it. Our systems of fat burning and running on empty have weakened. Give them a chance to get strong again, and they will help you get skinny.

So, starting tomorrow or whenever you start your plan, get more by doing less, and skip breakfast. **Your body is designed for this**. A basic part of this design is called stored breakfast, also known as body fat. Start to live off that brand!

And if you face a lot of criticism, get them to read this. Get them to study genetics, blood chemistry and ancient history. Now, if you thought reading this was hard to swallow, just wait for the next bit! In combination with this, it really gets fat moving.

GET THE SKINNY ON...

OMG 6 You can't burn fat if you have lots of energy in your system

OMG 5 Sleep uses up most spare energy throughout the night

OMG 4 When you wake up you're running on empty (good)

OMG 3 If you don't eat breakfast you'll eat body fat instead

OMG 2 We eat breakfast due to habit and commercial pressures

OMG 1 Our body isn't designed to wake up and instantly eat food

OMG ! Skip breakfast from now on!

SKINNY DIPPING

The bath tub. You probably think that it's just a place to have a soak, wash your hair, and forget all your worries. Well, if some of your worries are about being too fat or having thighs that make you cry, consider those worries lifted! How?

Water absorbs heat, *lots* of it, and it does it much quicker than air. If you happened to lay naked in an empty bath tub, apart from looking strange, you'd lose heat from your body, but lose it pretty slowly. Try it, it gets boring!

Now fill a bath with water that's the same temperature as the air. If you sit in that bath, your body would lose heat 25 times faster than the empty one. 25 times! Okay, so now you're thinking, '25 times, yay. Sorry, why do I care?'!

When you eat, some of your food calories are used to help your brain work, power your muscles, and generally keep you alive. Food energy is also used as fuel to keep your body at the right temperature. If you're warm, not much is needed.

The colder you get the more your body boosts heat production to keep you warm. As it does, some heat gets lost through skin. **When you're losing heat, you're losing energy. This energy has to come from somewhere.**

It all happens because of a weird type of tissue called BAT fat. That's **Brown Adipose Tissue** if you're about to enter a game show. Although it sounds like fat, it's actually a special bit of you that uses calories by *losing* them as heat.

We used to think that only babies had BAT fat, and that by the time they grew, it disappeared. Not so. Non-babies have some, especially those in colder countries, and you can boost yours too. It's time for you to become *Batgirl!*

The great thing about being exposed to cold, is that it raises your metabolism (the speed that you burn calories), *all day long*. The main thing that lowers your metabolic rate, is sleep. Sleep's downtime is important. Without it, we'd soon crash.

So, the best time to boost the metabolism is early as possible, and that means when you wake up. This way you'll get an increased metabolism for 12 - 15 hours. It's literally like being a more active person all day!

When this technique is combined with no breakfast and something else (next chapter), it causes such a jolt to the system, that it can kick-start even the most stubborn non-losers. **It takes a high amount of mental toughness**.

It also comes with **risks**. When you get into a cold bath, your body attempts to protect its core, that's all the important bits that keep you alive. Because of this, blood rushes there, pushing up your blood pressure slightly.

Also, the quick change in temperature forces the heart to work harder. **So, if you have a history of heart trouble, problems** with your blood pressure or diabetes, you must check with your doctor. Being dead is the wrong OMG.

Even if you are healthy, it's *extremely* important that you don't push harder than the guidelines. Being cold only works up to a point. Go beyond this, and you risk **hypothermia**. That's where the body gets *dangerously* cold.

You will need a few things. Ideally, all of them:

- A bath

- A plastic thermometer (or bath thermometer)

- A bath mat

- Something to time yourself with (e.g. phone or egg timer)

- Clothes for after

- Courage (lots!)

This is important. **You need the water cold enough to work, but not too cold that it makes you sick or scared**. Hardware stores sell thermometers. Get a plastic one. If you want, you can buy floating bath thermometers (often with a timer and alarm built-in).

So, how cold is cold? A warm bath is about 98–101 degrees Fahrenheit. **You need water that's between 59 and 68 degrees Fahrenheit**. The *feeling* of coldness varies depending on how much body fat you have (and where you have it).

Jumping straight into a cold bath is a bad idea. Most likely, you'll jump straight back out! And even if you could take it, it's best to let your body adapt slowly. Give it a week, and you'll probably stick with it.

Your goal is to do this every day for up to 15 **minutes**. This is enough time for the body to react and boost your metabolism for hours after. Longer times are *not* needed. It's potentially dangerous. And it's definitely boring!

Although our outsides are important to us, it's the insides that make your body happy. To keep them that way, when the body senses extreme cold, it tells the blood to leave the outside, and get to where it's needed. You may go pale (if you ever go blue, **stop immediately**).

GOODBYE THUNDER THIGHS

Cold baths have an unusual effect on the female lower body. Although fat may look the same all over, it's not. Some fat, especially in legs, is chemically stubborn. To lose this, it helps to get chemical stimulation.

We aren't sure why this is so, and research is still patchy. It's possible that because women can have children, stores of leg fat become determined to stick around just in case the calories are needed later.

To get your stubborn fat to play ball, we need to blast it with neurotransmitters and hormones, chemicals that *talk to* and *boost* cells. Two important ones are **adrenaline** (aka **epinephrine**) and its cousin **nor-adrenaline** (aka **nor-epinephrine**).

Cold bathing boosts both. Even if you can't take the full cold bathing experience, it's worth getting your legs cold. The legs contain a large number of cold receptors, so even just exposing them helps. A full skinny dip is obviously more powerful.

HOW TO TAKE A COLD BATH PROPERLY

Going straight into a full dip would be too much of a shock, and could temporarily take your breath away. This is not about self-punishment, so let's make it gradual and comfortable. Actually, comfortable is a lie!

A thermometer, timer and bath mat are important. One prevents you getting into water that's too cold, one stops you staying in the bath for too long, and the other stops you from slipping if you feel shaky. Get them.

ON YOUR MARKS

Run the bath! This will take about 6 to 10 minutes. You want the water level to reach your belly button when you're seated in the bath, with legs out in front and your upper body upright. Where's that bath mat? Put it in!

GET SET

You need the water temperature to be correct. In the beginning, you'll have no idea what's too cold or too warm unless you use the thermometer. It doesn't have to be exact, but **make sure it's not too cold**.

If it is, add a splash of warm water, swill it around, and check again. If it's too warm, and you're already using cold water by itself, it gets tricky. I know what you're thinking. Ice cubes!

Athletes use ice baths for about 2 minutes, usually to reduce severe muscle damage. Ice cubes are annoying. You have to make or buy them, carry them, and wait until they change the water temperature. Very dull!

Only those in super warm climates can't get water that's cold enough. I don't want to make this complicated. **All water, compared to the same air temperature, will help you lose calories fast**. Do your best with what you have.

HOLD ON

An egg timer, digital clock, watch or phone will all work the same. Make sure the alarm is loud enough. It's easy to lose track of time when you're out at sea! Place the timer somewhere you can see it.

GO

Step into the bath one foot at a time (written to warn twin-foot leapers!). Start the timer and stand still. You'll think, 'is *Venice* serious?'. Yes! Come on, don't wimp out. We've been to the moon and back (admittedly, in a warm space suit).

All of you, *Wavers*, *Blazers* and *Quakers*, will do the same warm-up (well I couldn't say 'cold-up'!). That means, all of you will stand like this for 2 minutes. Lift a foot out for a second and you'll feel heat. Put it back in!

I CAN'T FEEL MY LEGS

As your timer speeds towards 2 minutes, psych yourself up. You're going to sit down in the bath. If you sit slowly like an old man with a bad back, the cold shock to your behind might scare you! Sit down fast, like a kid playing musical chairs.

The first **shock** of cold will pass within a few seconds. And then comes the lapping of the water that *you* created! I advised you to sit down *fast*, not *dive!* As this water washes over the tops of your thighs and around your lower belly, you'll be tempted to quit. Hold on!

LAY BACK AND THINK OF *OMG*

Some of you will not go on to this next step, either because it's not part of your plan, or because you don't feel ready (or because you're scared). If you're in good health, and you've built up to it, you'll be okay.

So, you've had your legs in the water for almost 5 minutes. Some of you will be saying, 'can't I just stay like this?'! Of course, I'm not there to force you. But as I've said, the benefits are there if you want.

When you hit 5 minutes, *lean* back. The speed you do this is important. Don't go too fast (like sitting on musical chairs again) or you could hit your head, or create so much water movement that the cold shock keeps lapping at you for ages.

You need to go back at a medium speed. **This takes guts**. At *that* moment, you'll appreciate how much tougher your legs are, and realize that's why they need tons of stimulation to wake up and lose body fat.

Be strong. Just like when you first sat in the bath, the cold shock starts reducing as your body fires up its protective mechanisms. In the upper body, this takes a bit longer, and lots of cold pain receptors will scream, 'GET OUT NOW'!

After about 30 seconds, the cold shock feeling will reduce. It surges every so often as the water moves around and laps over your body. Water that's close to your skin is already warmer. New water is still cold, and you *will* feel the difference!

Depending on the size of the bath and the size of you, you'll either be covered with water or your knees may stick out. Let the back of your head just dip in. Most of your neck, and a bit of head. So what if your hair gets wet!

If you're too big for the bath, you'll have to find a way to make it work. Shift about so that overall, everything gets a bit of a shock. In the beginning, you'll try to keep still, but after a while, you'll actually enjoy the cold!

You'll notice that if you move your arms, water will rush up and around them, finding new places to wreak their cold chaos! **Eventually, your body will heat up so much of the water, that it will stop feeling so cold.**

If you've been a smart chick and used a thermometer, you might notice that the temperature you get out at, is 2 or more degrees higher than when you got in. And when it comes to getting out, everyone notices the strange feeling.

It will be a feeling of warmth, as your body has boosted heat production to the core, but continues to lose some through skin. If you're still cold and shivering, stay *calm*. Keep your focus, and get out of the bath carefully. You may be shaky.

Have something light to wear, or dress normally if you have plans for soon after. Listen up. **Don't have a warm bath or shower right after a cold one. This stresses your body to breaking point, and could cause you to faint**.

Get dressed and move around but don't go near the hot tap. Of course, a few hours later will be fine. I'm not talking about never washing your hands again! And for the curious ones, hot water doesn't undo the cold water effect. It's just painful.

Cold baths really boosts adrenaline and noradrenaline (aka epinephrine and norepinephrine). They stimulate your **Central Nervous System**. If you have a cold bath at night, these chemicals could stop you from sleeping.

If you're a girl at her time of the month, or as you get healthier, the feeling may be different. And the temperature of your city and your bathroom will affect how you feel. **Stay alert**, *change* things if you think it's necessary. You're the boss, even when you're naked!

This section may sound complicated, but after a few attempts, it's actually simple. The detail is to keep you safe, and to introduce the technique without frightening you. It's important to give it a try.

AND IF YOU REALLY CAN'T FACE IT

As I've said before, **you must never feel forced to do anything**. If it's too cold or if the bath idea scares you, don't give up the *entire* plan. The first step is to try a warm bath that's got a bit cooler than you'd normally like.

Even that helps, as all **water carries body heat away quickly, making your burn more calories**. If you can't even take that, wait until the weather is warmer, and give it another go. In the meantime, **do the rest of the plan**.

BRUSH AWAY YOUR TEARS

While you're in the bath, you might want to be distracted by listening to music or the radio. You might like to add in some **body brushing**. In our body, we have a kind of second blood-stream called a **lymphatic system**.

This system carries nutrients around the body. Cold baths already boost circulation, but body brushing can increase it more. Although research is limited, and hard to carry out, many find that body brushing really helps thighs.

And by help, I mean it improves their smoothness, and *might* even reduce that tear-jerking problem of cellulite. That's a whole other topic, but it's worth mentioning here. You need a body brush, and you always need to **brush *towards* the heart**.

In practical terms, you can't reach your lower legs (ankles to knees), because you'd have to lift out of the water. But you can gently brush from a just above your knees, up your thighs, come in at your waist, and over towards your heart.

You can brush your arms also. Starting at your wrists, brush up towards your elbow, along your upper arm, over your shoulder, and lightly across your chest. Make it a soft massage. Go smooth, constant and with a nice rhythm.

MAXIMUM TIME GOALS

WAVE

2 minutes standing

8 minutes seated

BLAZE

2 minutes standing

3 minutes seated

5 minutes laying back

QUAKE

2 minutes standing

3 minutes seated

10 minutes laying back

WATER TEMPERATURE GUIDE (FOR ALL)

Week 1 – aim for about 68° Fahrenheit

Week 2 – aim for about 66° Fahrenheit

Week 3 – aim for about 64° Fahrenheit

Week 4 – aim for about 62° Fahrenheit

Week 5 – aim for about 60° Fahrenheit

Week 6 – aim for about 59° Fahrenheit

THINK 15 / 15

DON'T get into a bath colder than 15° Celsius / 59° Fahrenheit

DON'T spend more than 15 minutes in a cold bath

HIT THE SHOWERS

So, what happens if you don't have a bath, is it the easy life for you? Of course not! If you're brave enough, and want to keep up with those skinny dippers, there's really only one option: hit the showers.

And remember, if you don't have a shower *or* bath, all is not lost. Anything that makes you feel cold, i.e. turning down the thermostat at home (or just walking around naked), is likely to help.

Yes, I admit, those things are pretty miserable! I just want you to know that the magic of cool isn't just available for those with nice homes. If any form of being cool isn't cool to you, take a chill pill, and do what you can.

Just before we go on, remember that everything you read about baths (I hope you read it, even if you don't own one), applies to showers too. **Check with your doctor first, and think safety at all times**.

Showers need to be approached differently to the bath. One simple reason is that if you get it wrong, it's easy to just step out of one! I would suggest that you still get your thermometer ready (at least once), a stopwatch, and have a shower mat to prevent slipping.

START LIKE A HOTTIE

Get into your *normal* shower temperature, stopwatch in hand (or on a nearby shelf). Start the clock, and stay in that for one minute. Yes, this is boring! If you're really smart, you'll use this minute to wash your hair (men only - girls, we *know* it takes you a whole evening!).

CHILL OUT

After a minute, turn the thermostat down a *notch*, making it cooler. If you have your thermometer, place it near the shower head (as your underarms start to complain at the thought of freezing), and keep it there for about 10 seconds. Check the temperature.

When you *start* your regular shower, it's likely to be around 86 to 100 degrees Fahrenheit (30 to 38 degrees Celsius), depending on what you find comfortable. **Your goal is to gradually bring the temperature down, once a minute, *until* it gets just under 68 degrees Fahrenheit (20 degrees Celsius).**

This takes considerable fiddling, I know! In practical terms, it may take 5 minutes, i.e. 5 lots of changing the temperature dial, to get close to 68 degrees Fahrenheit. **It may take less time, or it may take more, but regardless, it is important to do it slowly**.

Some of you could be thinking, "what's a *notch?*". Well, having not taken a shower at your place yet, I can't say. You will have to use your uncommonly good sense, and just work it out for yourself. Play about when you're *outside* the shower, see how you can control it.

ARE WE NEARLY THERE YET?

Once you get close to 68 degrees Fahrenheit, don't be tempted to make it any colder. In a cold bath, you can go a bit lower, but showers, depending on the size of the water droplets, can take your heat away *very* quickly. **Remember this**.

I would then advise you to stay in that cool stream for a *maximum* of 3 minutes. I realize that sounds like nothing. Just wait 'til you try it! And, I wouldn't go for 3 minutes immediately. **Spend a week to 10 days, building *up* to three minutes - start by mastering 30 seconds**.

The same guidelines for the baths apply here, perhaps even more so. **Do not warm yourself up with a warm shower - this is especially dangerous and could make you faint rapidly.** It's *much* safer to step out (at any time, if necessary), and wrap up in a robe, or clothing.

Repeating the entire sequence immediately is a bad idea, because rapidly changing your surface temperature back and forth confuses the brain, and shifts blood flow like tidal waves. **A second session, around 8 hours later (i.e. early evening), is safe, if you really want one**.

GET THE SKINNY ON...

OMG 6 Only use cold baths if you're in good health

OMG 5 Cold water makes us lose heat and this boosts calorie loss

OMG 4 Use the guidelines and let your body adjust slowly

OMG 3 Don't get in a bath colder than 59 degrees Fahrenheit

OMG 2 Don't spend more than 15 minutes in a cold bath

OMG 1 If you can't handle cold baths, don't give up everything

OMG ! Get a bath mat, thermometer and timer today!

BLACK GOLD

You now understand how a cold bath helps you burn more calories all day long. In the chapter after this, I'm going to talk about maximizing the benefits of that bath, by moving around. But before then, there's time for a quick drink!

Coffee. Nice? Yuk? Something that adults drink? Why care, we just want to burn fat! And coffee can help. It's nature's cheap and secret potion. If you use in the *right* way and at the *right* time, it *really* helps.

The secret is **caffeine**. Yes, just that. Caffeine boosts the central nervous system (like cold baths), the thing that controls most of your movement and electrical activity. When you have it on an empty stomach, it tells your body to burn fat much faster. How?

Caffeine makes fat cells open up and empty their fat into your bloodstream. From there, fat can be transported to your muscles. Once it arrives at your muscles, they use this liquid fatty fuel to power them. You get skinnier!

If you have caffeine and *don't* use this extra floating fat, you'll create problems. Left un-used, the fat would eventually react with air and form 'rust' in the arteries. Your heart definitely hates that.

But combine caffeine with something physical, and you get the opposite effect. You're emptying out bags of fat and burning the rubbish! Caffeine's effect lasts for 5 to 6 hours. That's a third of your hours awake.

Caffeine taken early in the day has plenty of time to lose its stimulating effect on the brain. Some people clear it from their system quickly, others slowly. As long as you're not having it past 4pm, it won't mess up your sleep.

The best forms of caffeine are liquids. Liquids are absorbed by the body quicker than solids, and also quicker than pills. This is ideal, as we then spend more time getting the benefit of what we're taking.

The most reliable place to find caffeine is, a **cup of coffee**. It's also in tea but at a lower concentration. To get the proper amount, you'd have to drink many cups, and in the process, you'd take in more water than a thirsty camel!

Because caffeine is well known for its effect on keeping us buzzing, you might already be planning to find it somewhere else. Hold on. Caffeine drinks that boost your energy are not suitable for fat burning. Why?

Well, you need the caffeine but you don't need the sugar, or artificial sweeteners. Remember, if there's gas in the tank, your body *won't* burn body fat. So, that means hardcore and possibly 'yuk' coffee for you!

No sugar and no milk. Either would tell your body that food's arriving. That would release a hormone called **insulin**, whose job is taking 'food deliveries' and shoving them into the warehouse (your fat cells and muscle cells).

If food is being brought *in*, your body knows that there's no point in letting food (body fat) *out*. It thinks, 'calories are arriving, so let's save our stored ones for a rainy day'. Sensible, but annoying!

So, black coffee it is. Artificial sweeteners don't have calories, but even their fake sweetness convinces taste buds into thinking food is on its way. They speak to the brain, which gets insulin up, and all your fat cells have a siesta! **Avoid all sweeteners**.

Black coffee might not be your favorite drink, and it might taste worse when too hot. Perhaps make some when the bath's running, and let it cool while you're splashing around. By the time you get out, you might even appreciate the warmth!

If you really can't stand the taste of coffee, buy caffeine pills. They're slower to dissolve than liquid coffee (BTW, capsules are faster than tablets), but at least you'll know exactly how much caffeine you're getting.

A cup of coffee has about 100 milligrams (mg) of caffeine, with drip coffee being slightly stronger than instant. Just so you know, a cup of tea contains 40 mg, a can of cola the same, and an energy drink usually has about 80mg.

A caffeine pill could contain 200mg. **Have up to 200mg caffeine per morning**. More would encourage trips to the toilet, and make you shaky too. Super high doses cause sleep trouble and even irregular heart beats (not good).

The combination of no breakfast, a cold bath and a caffeine boost is powerful. When you follow these methods with the next section, you'll burn fat faster than ever before. It sounds complicated, but it's actually easy to get into.

Although coffee has been around for years, it doesn't mean that it can't be an effective fat burner. It's all about *timing*. Most people don't use coffee like a drug. They drink it, but they don't move.

Mixed with milk and sugar or sweeteners, plus a donut or three, coffee turns into a useless drug! It really has a chemical *Jekyll and Hyde* split personality. That's why it goes undiscovered by those looking for fat loss.

GET THE SKINNY ON . . .

OMG 6 Caffeine boosts your central nervous system

OMG 5 This makes you burn more body fat as a fuel

OMG 4 A cup of coffee is the easiest way to get caffeine

OMG 3 Caffeine won't work if you have calories with it

OMG 2 If you hate black coffee, use caffeine pills

OMG 1 Have up to 200mg of caffeine in the morning

OMG ! Caffeine works so use some properly tomorrow!

MOVE OVER EXERCISE

Exercise is just *so* 2011! For many people, the 'E' word gets a bad image, and sometimes, it's easy to see why. We get introduced to exercise in school, where it tends to be serious, boring, and sometimes even used as a punishment!

Forget all that. Your body doesn't care about 'exercise' either. Your body just likes to keep moving. Scientists who have carefully followed 'naturally slim' people and their daily physical habits, have known this all along.

They noticed that those who moved most, happened to be the skinniest. Those who hardly moved, tended to be fatter. Of course, it's just one element, but it's important. Scientists described their discovery as 'the fidget factor'.

Obviously, this strange phrase didn't really catch on with the public. So for the past 20 years, aware that people were sometimes scared of the 'E' word, scientists came up with an apparently more appealing word. Activity.

Activity? You can see why scientists are better off discovering and not explaining! It's possibly worse than 'exercise', as for most people, it doesn't clearly tell us what to do. Leave 'activity' for something done in a kindergarten!

I'm going to suggest something else, and I promise it won't start with a vowel. This word describes the truth behind what scientists discovered, and it simplifies the only important thing we need to remember. **Movement**.

You might be thinking, 'is that it?'. Yeah! Don't laugh at it being too simple, because the simplicity is its beauty. Business loves to sell you complicated stuff. Complicated things sound like a magic formula. **Your body doesn't believe in diet superstitions**.

It believes this. Every time you ask it to move a muscle, even just to blink, it takes energy. Don't worry, I'm not suggesting you blink your way to being skinny, because that would just get the wrong kind of OMG reaction!

Movement requires energy, and that's literally all your body knows. That energy can come from the calories in new food (e.g. refrigerator, store, drive-thru), or from the calories in old food (e.g. thigh fat, butt fat, *any* body fat!).

Think about the device you might be reading this on. At some point, it runs low on power, and you attach a cable and re-charge it. Movement is our way to run down the batteries (calories) on purpose. It's part of a natural process.

No? Okay, remember the car and gas analogy from before. We said that getting fuel at a gas station was like eating food. And that our blood, liver and muscles are like a car's gas tank, containing the energy from any recent food.

But there's more. Stored body fat is like a spare hidden gas tank. Well, body fat is rarely hidden! And this emergency supply actually contains more fuel than everything else combined. Each pound of body fat contains 3500 calories.

Three and a half thousand? 3-5-0-0. Told you the body wasn't expecting to find food easily! Now you can appreciate how important it is to make sure that this supply of stored energy gets used (i.e. breakfast is for wimps)!

So, what's the best way to tap into this huge supply? To do whatever makes you move! Am I being silly? No! This is just one of the 4 basic ideas I'd like you to think about. They'll help you decide what type of movement is good for you:

MOVING IS LOSING

If your body is moving, it's happy. And it doesn't know where you are when you do it. You could be running in the street or running in a gym, and your body wouldn't spot the difference. It just knows the important thing. Whether you are moving.

This idea will help you realize that when you can't do your favorite form of moving, you don't need to get upset. Try something else for that day. Your body only gets upset if you don't do anything at all. Simple.

MOVE MORE FINGERS AND TOES, BURN MORE CALORIES

And I don't mean *just* move your fingers and toes, although they help! I mean, **the more muscles you use at any time, the more**

calories you will burn. This idea is so logical, it's truly amazing how many people seem to do the opposite.

For example, if you do sit-ups, you're using a *small amount of muscle*. Therefore, you're only able to burn a *small amount of energy*. Even if you do thousands, you're still burning tiny amounts of energy each time. The fat over your abs won't change.

But, let's say you sit down on a chair, and stand up. That uses *lots* of muscles. That's right, our favorite game of *musical chairs* burns lots of calories! So, in any minute, the more muscle you move, the higher the calories you can burn.

Let me give you a better example than party games. Cycling uses your legs, big muscles which use a decent amount of calories. But walking uses arms, shoulders, stomach, chest, back *and* your legs! **More muscles equals more calories**.

You have the power to estimate what movements will work well for you. You may also realize that using your arms to hold onto a treadmill means burning less than you could. And that the crazier you dance, the more you burn!

FASTER DOESN'T MEAN BETTER

Technically speaking, if you move your muscles more times per minute, you will be burning more calories per minute. And, faster movements boost your calorie burning after exercise.

But, faster movements also make it hard for your heart, lungs and muscles. To move fast, your body needs to suck in lots of oxygen, and absorb it quickly. Your heart races, you breathe much quicker and your muscles might scream.

To get lots of oxygen into your body, you need to be fit. The fitter you get, the more your body can cope with this high-speed moving. But the really important question is, do you need to be fit to burn calories? No.

For example, whether you run, walk or crawl a mile, you'll still burn about the same number of calories. Back to our car analogy! Visualize two flags, 1 mile apart. To drive from one flag to another always takes the same amount of gas.

The only slight difference, is that if you drive fast (move your body fast), you heat up a bit more, and this extra bit of heat means you'll burn an extra bit of gas (calories) later. But it's actually a small difference in terms of total fat burning.

Moving fast makes you *fit*, but we're here for *fat*. If you move fast, you may burn less calories overall than moving slower and going for longer.

Normal speed moving, especially if you're new to physical stuff, also helps you avoid feeling too tired *after*. For some of you, if your intensity is super high, you might crash and hardly move. And that's worse than doing nothing!

As you lose fat, your fitness will start to get better. And eventually, you will be able to go faster. When you can move lots of muscle fast and for a long time, you'll use huge amounts of energy. Until then, take a chill pill and *stroll!*

DO WHAT MAKES YOU HAPPY

This is the *most* important thing. You can get all the other stuff, but if the way you move doesn't suit your groove, you're not going to do it at all! So, find what excites you (or if you really hate moving, find what depresses you least!).

Some people are suited to fun forms of movement, like dance. Others prefer being able to see progress, and use machines or electronics that display how they're doing. **The only important thing is if a form of movement suits *you*.**

Your body might be suited to a particular kind. For example, people with bad feet might prefer to use a cross-training machine, and those who get too hot might only enjoy swimming. Do movement that suits you.

MOVEMENT THAT USE LOTS OF MUSCLE

Walking or Running

Dancing (especially dancing crazily!)

Rowing machine

Cross trainer machine

Workout DVD (only if it has movement in it!)

MOVEMENT THAT USES SOME MUSCLE

Cycling

Step machine

Seated exercise bike

MOVEMENT THAT USES LITTLE MUSCLE

Skipping

Trampoline

Sit-ups or crunches

JUST MOVE IT

So you've got up, had a cold bath, a cup of coffee and you've left breakfast on the shelf. Now you need to move! But how much do you need to do? Well, a decent chunk during the 6 weeks, but maybe not as much as you thought.

The first **period of m**ovement, let's call it **pom 1**, must really be designed to take advantage of the morning. That means picking the most effective type of movement for you, and doing it for the longest time that is practical.

The minimum time for pom 1 is 30 minutes. Although every minute spent moving in the morning will help you burn fat, a shorter time would really waste a golden opportunity. And 30 minutes sets the body up nicely for what comes later.

WAVE - pom 1 **30 minutes**

BLAZE - pom 1 **45 minutes**

QUAKE - pom 1 **45 minutes** (same as **BLAZE**, not a typo!)

Some might be wondering if you can do more than this. The amounts look neat, but they're not just to look pretty. They're designed to make you pretty! And they're amounts designed with other parts of the plan in mind.

But, if you want to do more, go for it. **Don't do more than 60 minutes for pom 1**. It might be difficult to schedule and could make you ill or bored. It could also affect the balance of what the rest of the plan has in store for you.

Going beyond 60 minutes does seem to cause problems. The longer we go, the more we subconsciously hold back on how hard we work. Your kind mind literally tries to protect the body from effort!

If you can, get outside in view of daylight to do your movement session. Natural daylight, especially morning light from 8 to 9 a.m. resets your internal body clock and raises Vitamin D production. Light can even boost happy hormones!

And here's a note for the super hungry in the morning types. If you wake up *desperate* for food and think, 'no *way* can I go out without breakfast', think again.

Soon as you start moving, the body starts to focus on that, and will dampen down your appetite. Give it a go.

VERY IMPORTANT ADVICE FOR AFTER POM 1

When you've completed your moving around in the morning, what you do next is very important. **You must not eat for 3 hours**. Of course you can drink water, but that's it. No sports drinks, snacks, bars, shakes, and certainly no breakfast!

When you make the body move, it causes many good chemical changes. **You will keep burning body fat until you eat**. And that doesn't mean never eat again! That would end in disaster. It will make more sense in the next section.

Just remember that as soon as you eat, your body *senses* it. It will then immediately stop burning body fat and shift over to burning whatever you feed it. You'll eventually eat, but why not fat burn to the max?

WHAT ABOUT WEEKENDS?

If your body heard that question it would say, 'what about weekends?'. If *you* don't appreciate someone singing about *Friday*, you can't expect your body to! Humans *invented* Monday to Friday to make our lives more ordered. And we invented the weekend too!

So what does this mean? It means that if a technique works, there's nothing to stop you from using it every day, *including* weekends. **This is where many plans go wrong**. They suggest 'days off'. Nice in theory. But we don't do theory!

I could pretend and say that days off are necessary for your mind. But I won't. **During these 6 weeks, there aren't days off**. If you get sick, rest up. But if you're not, you're simply stopping due to the letters of the alphabet!

In fact, many of the benefits in this book, work well for 24 hours. It's no accident. Sleep tends to reset stuff. All this doesn't mean that you're stuck on a plan for life, but for a short period of time, you've got to make proper changes.

Use every technique in the book, every day. There are times when *stuff* gets in the way of plans, and that's cool. As long as you admit that you're stopping because of life and not because you think 'hey, Saturdays don't count'!

And don't think pom 1 is an only child! It has a brother and sister who share first names, pom 2 and pom 3! They're little brothers and sisters in comparison, but they're important, and they need a separate bedroom (chapter). Until then.

GET THE SKINNY ON...

OMG 6 Your body just cares about movement

OMG 5 Do 30 to 60 minutes of movement in the morning

OMG 4 Find movement that involves lots of muscle

OMG 3 But make sure that it's something you really enjoy

OMG 2 Use movement every day unless you're ill

OMG 1 You don't need to get fit to lose fat

OMG ! After your first movement session don't eat for 3 hours!

MIND THE GAP

'Eat frequently' is a phrase you'll hear experts say often. Perhaps by choosing the word 'frequently', their advice is meant to sound scientific. Unfortunately, some translate 'eat frequently' into 'eat more'!

And this is exactly what many do. We've been encouraged to believe that each time we eat, we boost our metabolism and our chances of losing weight. This is very wishful thinking, and it's wrong.

It's all based, *on a theory*. When you eat, some of a meal's calories are burned by the digestive process itself. So, in theory, by eating lots of small meals *more often*, you lose extra calories, from digesting *more often*.

Some scientists have turned creative, using the words 'graze' and 'gorge'. They encourage us to 'graze' throughout the day, perhaps like a cow innocently plucking at grass in a sunny field. Hey mister scientist, we're not cows!

And they have a warning word, 'gorge'. Don't eat big meals or you'll be a naughty pig! Hardly subtle persuasion. So are they right, does 'gorging' food mean that you're greedy and have no manners?

Not at all. For a start, cows can be pigs at times, and pigs generally get a bad rap anyway! Really, this commonly used graze

82

and gorge mentality isn't how most people apply the 'eat more frequently' advice.

Let's say you normally ate 3000 calories per day, in three meals of 1000 each. Then you get told to eat small meals more frequently. If you're like most people, you wouldn't naturally divide your meals into 6 perfect servings of 500 calories each.

Any shift in eating habits is tough, but cutting calories from 1000 to 500 per meal and sticking to it is very unlikely. Most people tend to reduce their calories at each meal by a much smaller amount.

You might reduce calories from 1000 to 750 per meal, but because there's now 6 meals of that, you're eating 4500 in total! **That's a 50% increase over what you would have had before listening to the 'eat frequently' theory.**

It's true, *some* of a meal's calories are used up by digestion. But it's nowhere near enough to recommend that we 'graze'! Science often gets too excited with theory, and members of the public become their guinea pigs.

We'd all benefit from eating better food, in smart amounts, and *less* frequently. I realize that the idea of eating three meals per day seems old fashioned. Guess what, being fat is a modern fashioned problem!

The scientists who recommended this frequent eating, forgot to think about the bigger picture. Our genetics. And I mean, why we have stores of body fat in the first place. Listen up white coats, it's time to go back to school!

In the days before pizza could be ordered online and refrigerators could keep ice cream cold in summer, we had to find our food wherever it existed. I'm talking about our cousins here, the cavemen and cavewomen (cave pets too).

They never knew when food was going to turn up, which I'm sure you'll agree is pretty scary. And obviously, not everyone is skillful enough to hunt an animal or find luscious vegetation. So, Mother Nature gave us body fat.

Now before you curse her, think about it. Walking around for hours, searching for food *takes* energy. And where would we find it, when we're out looking for some in the first place? Body fat! This was nature's idea of balance.

You could think of body fat in this ancient sense, as another food backpack we carry on big missions. Remember, each pound of body fat contains 3500 stored calories. This energy is stored, but it's not supposed to be stored forever!

Body fat exists to give us energy when we're not taking any in. This can only happen in gaps between meals. The more often you eat, the shorter the gaps get.

The biggest gap is from your last meal at night, to the first meal a few hours after you've done pom 1. This could be up to 16 hours, and during this time, constant fat burning takes place. Your body *loves* this.

MEALS STOP YOU GETTING HUNGRY

At first, that subtitle seems obvious. If you're hungry and you eat something, your appetite goes away. It's so obvious, that for years, both scientists and anyone else who eats, actually forgot to investigate deeper into why it happens.

Wait no more. When you eat, your body senses that food is coming in, and it releases a chemical called **leptin** (the Greek word for *skinny*). Leptin tells our brain that we've eaten enough. It shouts at us to 'STOP'!

Got it? Let's make sure...with another car analogy! **Leptin is like a fuel gauge**. When you fill up with gas (start eating), it senses this. When you've got enough gas (food) it says, 'you can take the nozzle out now'. You stop eating.

This is why it's bad to eat fast. Our gas gauge takes 20 minutes to assess how much you've filled up on. Sometimes, we wolf food down so quickly that by the time the body works out what's going on, you've already eaten an entire feast!

Back to the point. **Meals raise leptin better than snacks, shutting off appetite for longer**. Other things also reduce appetite, and I talk about these in their own sections. For now, it's important to understand that meals are best.

There's more. **New research shows that leptin not only tells appetite when to calm down, but it tells the metabolism to rev up**. It's logical. Once leptin senses that you've got enough fuel, it tells your body to start using it.

Controlling your appetite is critical. Food is the main factor that affects our weight, and appetite is the main factor that affects our food choice. Controlling your appetite doesn't mean starvation! We just need it to work properly.

If you have problems controlling your appetite, the main reason is that you eat too often. Stop today. Put it down! **Eating less often is the first way to train your appetite**. You'll soon notice how few people eat three times per day.

Three *meals* per day is ideal. It's plenty for getting variety into our diet, it's spaced out enough to let us burn body fat in between meals, and it's social too. Eating meals together, not snacks, is one of life's greatest joys.

By the way, don't get put off by the word. I realize that some of us have a bad feeling when we see or hear 'meal'. It could mean being forced to sit at a table, eating stuff you hate, or it's that thing that *always* interrupts your important phone calls!

As with 'exercise', your body doesn't understand 'meal', so be cool. When you see the 'm' word, it just means eating (or drinking) something for your body. Give it any name, just do it three times per day!

If you're new to this concept of eating meals, and only three times per day, get ready for an argument with your brain and stomach! **Most of us eat 10 or more times per day**. Think I'm exaggerating? See how often a calorie passes your lips.

To help you get used to this new gorge pattern (gorge makes you gorgeous!), forget about what's *in* your meals for a few days, just get used to having them. **Get used to having longer gaps between eating**.

In terms of spacing meals apart, the obvious way is to divide them equally, but this is often not practical for life. Be flexible, go with the flow. Your first meal will probably be around the traditional lunchtime. You get breakfast at last!

The timing for the other two meals are up to you. **I suggest that your last meal is about two hours before you expect to sleep**. In the beginning this could be difficult, especially if you're used to eating right up to nodding off!

If that is you, *gradually* increase the final gap between your last meal and sleep. It might take you a week, but it's important. You don't want to go to bed feeling hungry, because you might wake up craving food. Not good.

But you also don't want to go to bed feeling full. A meal takes time to digest, though I'm not concerned about digesting the food itself. Undigested food is uncomfortable, but it digests eventually. Avoiding being full is crucial for another reason.

In the first few hours after you sleep, your body releases growth hormone. This natural chemical is super powerful. It boosts other good chemicals, makes your skin smooth and firm, reduces body fat and tones muscle. All while you dream!

Research has discovered that **this boost of growth hormone only occurs if your blood sugar is low**. So that means that it can only show up when there's not much food in your system. Plan for that 2 hour gap.

By now, you understand there's no such thing as a healthy snack. All that 'healthy snack' stuff you hear (e.g. dried fruit, nuts, bars, yogurts and fruit, *whatever*), *none of it* is healthy between meals. **Ditch the snack, love the gap!**

GET THE SKINNY ON...

OMG 6 Eating frequently make us eat more of everything

OMG 5 You only burn fat in the long gaps between meals

OMG 4 If you eat often you won't burn fat often

OMG 3 The overnight gap is long so use it well

OMG 2 Meals raise leptin and that controls appetite

OMG 1 There's no such thing as a healthy snack

OMG ! Start eating three spaced apart meals per day!

APPETITE FOR SUCCESS

As we've seen, the combo of skipping breakfast, skinny dipping, coffee, movement and gaps between meals makes sense. We also know that meals themselves are the way to go, but the question is, what to put in them?

This book is about making you look great, and the biggest thing to ruin your chances, is an appetite that always gets the better of you. Choosing what to eat seems to get more confusing the more we read, but some stuff always works.

One of the most basic things you need to know about, is **protein**. The name comes from the Greek, meaning *of first importance*. They really picked a good word for it, as protein affects your appetite, and much more.

PROTEIN - STUFF FOR BOYS (APPARENTLY)

Ask most people what protein is, and they'll say 'meat'. That's it, protein done! On a good day, someone might be more daring and say 'chicken', 'pepperoni' or 'steak'. Those are just descriptions of *where* you find protein.

But what is it? Everything in the universe is made from atoms, the smallest things we've found. Stick a few atoms together, and they make an element. Combine a few of those and we have an **amino acid**. Boring stuff almost done!

Think of amino acids as jewelry beads. String some beads together, and you make a necklace. And that my friend, is protein, a necklace. Now, for a girl to be at her best, I think you'll agree, she needs a lot of necklaces!

And it's the same with the human body. Our skin, hair, nails, organs, hormones, even our *thoughts*, are made from lots of necklaces getting together in one area. Drain out our water, and our body is over 50% necklaces. I mean 50% protein!

To keep our collection going, we need lots of beads. Humans can't make them, so we must find them. Where? Why the mall of course! We find beads and ready-made necklaces in food. And just like stores in the mall, some are better than others.

To make anything human, we just need 8 types of bead. Maybe imagine them as colors of the rainbow, plus one more. Eat enough of these 8 super beads (please, *don't* eat bead beads!), and you're making at least half of your body happy.

These 8 super beads are called the **essential amino acids**. They're essential because without them, we would eventually die. As I said, a girl needs necklaces! Because so much of us is made from protein, we need to keep topping up supplies.

Like us, animals are made from necklaces and beads. If you eat them, you're stealing (eating) their supply of necklaces. We used to assume that meat was our only source of protein. Now we know that's not strictly correct.

Nature knows that some of us are awful hunters, or don't like hunting at all (i.e. vegetarians). So, even non-animal foods contain beads. Beans, nuts, and even vegetables contain some, but you must try to eat a nice variety.

So, we know that **half of our body is made from protein**. In recent times, science has discovered that protein has other useful qualities, and one is super important. **Protein helps control our appetite**. And it makes complete sense.

Half of us is breaking down *constantly.* Pull a hair out, sit, stand, even just rub a few skin cells off by putting your jeans on, and you're losing protein. Protein loss is part of life and it never stops. We must attempt to replace this.

And because we can't magic it up, we have to eat some. Your body is well aware of this. Although scientists don't know why, **I am certain that the body looks out for protein, just as leptin looks out for calories**.

We definitely know that **if you eat enough protein, the body quickly reduces your appetite, and keeps it low for hours**. It does this better than any other nutrient, including fiber, which is known for doing that.

The most important part of any meal, is making sure that it contains protein. If your meal doesn't have enough, you'll be hungrier than you need to, and you will overeat. You're also ignoring the stuff needed to make great hair, skin and nails.

When selecting a protein food, the goal is to get something that's mostly protein. It's unlikely that you can get pure protein, but *aim* for it. Aim for *mostly protein*. Never count the calories or fat in your source of protein. Just get protein!

THE SOURCE OF THE SAUCE

Be careful about your protein source being covered in sauce. In seconds, a liquid can turn a perfectly healthy choice, into something amazingly wrong. This is how fast-food companies ruin great products, and your waistline!

To give you an idea of what I mean, consider this. A piece of chicken, cooked in virtually any way, will mostly be protein. And for our purposes, that's great. But add a sauce, and I mean almost any sauce, and you've changed it completely.

That plate now probably has a third of its calories from carbs. And that's before you've officially added carbs at all! You'd be surprised what's in most sauces. Tell me, would you pour soft drinks over chicken? These sauces are worse!

Even traditional coverings, like breadcrumbs, tend not to be so traditional any more. I have seen at least one brand of breadcrumbs that doesn't contain any bread! I'm not saying bread is a good thing, but come on!

I'm not talking about natural coverings like the skin on a chicken. I'm talking about the man-made (woman-made more likely!) stuff. Go for simple seasonings like black pepper, olive oil or balsamic vinegar.

Gravy, mayo and ketchup quickly ruin the 'mostly protein' vibe! Even fast-food restaurants have good foods ruined by sauces. But order without sauce, or add your own, and often their food is excellent. Yes, even *McDonald's*.

GOOD PROTEINS FOR NON-VEGETARIANS

All meats including chicken, turkey, beef and lamb, fish including cod, tuna, haddock and salmon, and eggs (boiled, scrambled, omelet).

GOOD PROTEINS FOR VEGETARIANS

Plain yogurt (not 'low-fat'), tofu (soy), *Quorn* (some products only), chick peas, lentils, peanuts, almonds, most seeds and whey protein (a powder from health stores).

LIVING ON POWDERS

For some people, either those on the move, or vegetarians who are sometimes stuck for choice, protein powders are a miracle in a tub (or sachet). If you use any of these, get ready for some opposition. Some say, 'they're not real food'.

They're completely wrong. In the case of whey protein, it's made from milk. It's then pushed through a filter. What's left is an almost pure protein that's absorbed by humans better than any other type.

This particular powder is so useful, it's even used in hospitals. For example, in burns patients who have lost lots of their own protein (e.g. their skin), whey helps speed recovery. It's suitable for many, including those who can't digest milk itself.

Of course, it may not come with the iron found in meat, or the special fats found in fish, but they don't come with certain nutrients that whey comes with. And besides, most of your nutrients will come from vegetables, and some from fruit.

There are other powders, such as soy protein powder, and even one made from peas. These aren't as well absorbed as whey protein, but they're still real food. **Ignore those who make a snap judgment if you use powdered supplements**.

If you're going to use one, keep it simple and buy just for the protein content. Don't get caught up in hype. Buy from an old company, and make sure that it meets everything from the following checklist:

- 70 grams or more protein per 100 grams (3.5 oz) of dry powder

- 10 grams or less carbs per 100 grams (3.5 oz) of dry powder

- Doesn't contain *Aspartame* or *Acesulfame K*

HOW MUCH PROTEIN?

The technical answer is neither interesting nor easy to remember! Most people don't like having to read food labels, and when you find a food without one, you're stuck anyway. So, it's time to get totally non technical, and totally practical.

HALF TIME

Hopefully by now, you're already keen on eating meals, and if so, at least some of the time you'll be using a plate. If you're not using a plate, you'll just have to imagine one! Next, I want you to mentally divide that plate in half. Easy.

And on that half, you put down your protein. 'Half?', you scream! Yes, half. As I said, it's an easy way to divide a plate, and if it's easy, you'll stick to it. Plus a little coincidence is that both you and your plate are half protein!

You may think this means you're on a half protein diet. No way. Protein foods aren't all protein, so even if half of your plate estate is protein, it won't be a 50% protein diet. Other plate invaders will change it from 20 to 40%. Anyway, forget numbers.

The main thing, is that you **fill one side of your plate with protein at *every* meal**. If at times your source of protein is a liquid, and you're not sure about how much that works out to be, use up to one large cup of it (12 ounces or 350 ml, or about 20g of protein).

You don't have to fill a plate so that protein spills over the sides! One more thing; make sure that the protein half isn't overtaken by other foods. Remember the ancient Greek definition, *of first importance*. We'll get to what's on the other half in a while.

I realize that this half plate of protein might be tricky to start with. Stick at it. Your first meal is especially important. Why? **Movement can boost appetite, so your first meal is your first roadblock against it**. Get protein.

PROTEIN: THE HOT GUY

Protein increases heat production in the body. It's hard for the body to process, taking a few extra calories to do so. The

95

effect is small, similar to eating frequent meals, but it's more than you get from carbs or fat, and you need protein anyway.

Most people have been eating very low protein diets for a long time. Protein is the most expensive type of calorie for food companies, so most of our food is carbs and some fat. **When you start increasing your protein, you may feel warmer**.

Protein, the hot guy of all the food types, is just doing its thing. In fact, it's the perfect diet guy. He makes you warm, he makes your skin, hair and nails look great, and he even stops you looking for other guys (he reduces your appetite!).

GET THE SKINNY ON...

OMG 6 Half of your body is protein and it breaks down constantly

OMG 5 You can't make protein so you must eat it daily

OMG 4 Dietary protein helps control your appetite

OMG 3 Dietary protein will make your hair, skin and nails amazing

OMG 2 Find proteins that don't come with many carbs

OMG 1 Have protein with all of your meals

OMG ! Eat proteins you like and fill half your plate with them!

THE SECOND HALF

Right, you've got an idea about half of your plate, stick some protein on it! The other side of your plate is the tricky half. Most good scientists can't deny the facts on protein. But almost everyone has an opinion on everything else.

Why are there so many arguments? Is it because people are trying to promote certain diets and diet products? Perhaps it's because each group really believes their way is best? Or are we confused by the constantly changing science?

It's a mixture of all three. So, what's a girl to do? Well I'm not interested in old fashioned opinions or pushing special products. And I'm not confused by the science. I am interested in facts, and only the facts that work.

CARBS

Carbohydrates is their full name, but hey in today's world, we definitely know them well enough to call them **carbs**. In fact, carbs now completely dominate our stores, refrigerators, thoughts, and way too many of our behinds!

There are many types of carbs. I could describe all of them (stop sighing!) but I'm not (stop yaying!). I am going to steal the useful science stuff. Carbs can be made from one bit, two bits joined, lots of bits joined, or lots and lots of bits joined!

What are those bits? **Sugars**. Most carbs we eat are made from one sugar, or two sugars joined up. Sugar doesn't only mean the white stuff you put in your coffee. Actually, we don't do sugar in coffee!

Okay, it's time for you to hear it. **Humans don't need carbs**. That's zero, as in none. Nothing! If you stopped having carbs right now, you wouldn't die. In fact, you'd live a long and skinny life. Might be boring though. Okay, deep breath.

As you already know, we need protein, or we would eventually fall apart. And as you'll discover, fats need to come along for the ride too. But carbs? We don't need them. How could a tasty thing like carbs not be necessary?

FUEL FOR THOUGHT

Two things in our body need fuel. Our organs, including our brain, and our muscles. They can both run on **glucose**, a one 'bit' sugar. We can get glucose by eating carbs and turning them into it. And we can actually do this with any type of carbs.

Donut carbs turn into glucose, carrot carbs turn into glucose, and if you lick the back of a postage stamp, even that glue turns into glucose! Glucose, also known as **blood sugar** (or just think **carbs**) is our body's most common drink.

But somehow, Mother Nature knew that there might be times when we couldn't get carbs. Maybe she knew that most of us weren't good at climbing banana trees, or even finding them! And maybe she knew, that bad weather often wipes carbs out.

So, she gave us another way to find energy. Muscles, as you may recall, can burn body fat. And then, there's our liver. Even without carbs, it can still fix your brain a drink. It can turn protein from food into glucose. Party trick one.

For party trick two, the liver takes a bit of fat and protein from your plate, plus a lot of fat from your butt, and turns it into a fuel called **ketones**. It uses this to power itself and gives some to our brain, which also runs brilliantly on it.

For millions of years, this is exactly how most humans got their energy. They simply lived off their own belly fat, behind or thighs, and got a few more cals from the fat and protein they ate. Finding and eating carbs was rare.

Now, these ketone guys only show up when our carb intake drops low. For example, they show up in the morning after a long sleep and in long gaps between meals. Or, if you simply keep carbs out of the house! **Ketones show, when carbs don't.**

Let me summarize, because the science can sound tricky to start with. Your body can run on 3 main types of fuel.

glucose - made mostly from carbs

body fat - made from wherever you have it!

ketones - made mostly *from* your body fat (wherever you have it!)

Most girls only ever burn carbs for energy. Wherever there's 'western' food, there are high carbs, and that blocks the chance of running on ketones. But if you've never heard of ketones, surely they don't matter?

OH YES THEY DO! Relax, I'm not about to suggest a zero carb diet. That's got a zero chance of success. Most of us like to go out and eat socially, and our world is covered with carbs from wall to wall. Don't lick too many postage stamps now!

So, was my ancient history lesson just for fun? Nope! This ketone system exists inside *all* of us, and it's such a big clue that we can't ignore it. While zero carbs are not practical for the modern cavewoman, we must avoid the opposite.

We must teach our body to be less carb dependent. 99 out of 100 experts see ketones as some kind of emergency back-up system. These are the distant family relations of those who recommended not sailing too far, just in case you fell off the planet. Be the 1 who sails on, and realizes that in fact, **carbs are meant to be our back-up**. It's a big shift in thinking. Huge.

We are literally designed to live off our body fat stores throughout the majority of the day. We're not designed to walk around attached to a grocery store. We *are* the grocery store! To access our own store, total carbs must be low.

So, what's the right amount? Well, it does vary from person to person, depending on factors like your genes, and how healthy your muscles are. I realize that you want numbers! And for that, you'll have to count numbers too.

So far, I've given you no reason to count anything. And you'll never need to count calories, percentage fat, or even protein (just have half a plate). But when it comes to carbs, at least for 6 weeks, you'll need some help.

NEVER EAT MORE THAN 4 IPHONES (OR 4 BLACKBERRYS)

Is that unusual advice, or do you already know that plastic is hard to digest? Bear with me here, there's some logic in the madness! When it comes to setting an *upper limit* for carbs, we all could do with a simple picture in our head.

Just like us, our phones have been growing. *Blackberrys* and *iPhones* nicely match the upper limit for a portion of mainly carb food. Don't have one of these phones? They take up the same plate space as a DVD disk.

On your plate, imagine you had two of these phones side by side, plus two more on top of them. **This is the upper limit of any carbs-based food that you'd ever need**. It's roughly the size of 10 stacked DVD disks.

Does this sound ridiculous and unscientific? It's definitely unscientific, but it's definitely not ridiculous. Once you're beyond 6 weeks, you need a guide. Critics can laugh, but success comes from practicality. Fact.

In this amount, I'm referring to foods that are mainly carbs. **Never count vegetable carbs**. Vegetables are super healthy plants, containing many nutrients, little sugar, much fiber, rich taste, good fat, variety, color and even a splash of protein.

Eat vegetables without any* restriction, from day 1 of doing _Six Weeks To OMG_, until your last day alive!

But before you can guess carbs by imagining them as phones or DVDs, you need a bit more precision. And for a while you'll need to glance at labels. It's easy. You just need one number. And you need to track it for 6 weeks.

CARBS DOWN YOUR THROAT

In a nutshell, this is _the_ most important figure for your figure. It really is! I'm not asking you to calculate a fancy percentage. **You simply need to know how many grams of carbs you're putting in your mouth (ignoring vegetables).**

Almost everything we eat today has a food label, and if it doesn't, _Google_ will easily find out what it's made of. You're not counting your calories, your protein, your fat, or your veg-etables. You're just keeping an eye on your pure carbs.

Once you've mastered this for 6 weeks, with a variety of carb foods, you'll be able to feel limitless. And of course, you'll always have the four _iPhones_ or _Blackberrys_ guide as a visual reminder. Or 10 DVDs. That's DVD disks, not DVD cases!

So, coming up are the suggested amounts for the 6 weeks. Some of you might find getting these figures easy, and others might find it hard, at least to start with. If you go over them on one day, the world won't end.

WAVE - up to **120 grams** of non-vegetable **carbs** per day

BLAZE - up to **90 grams** of non-vegetable **carbs** per day

QUAKE - up to **60 grams** of non-vegetable **carbs** per day

It's super crucial that you get *under* these daily carb totals. Don't panic about having too many carbs in one meal. It's far more important to just get under your daily total. If you do that, you'll keep your daily insulin level low too.

Need an insulin refresher? It's the hormone that your body releases when you eat carbs. The brain scoops up what it needs, and then insulin takes the leftovers and puts them into muscle or fat cells.

When you're releasing insulin, it means 'food is being stored'. And when the body is *storing* food, you can't *release* food (i.e. body fat) at the same time. It's one or the other. Want it as simple as possible? This is an example of a great Monday:

Monday's carbs low = Monday's insulin low = Monday's body fat burning high

TOTAL DOMINATION

Keeping the *total* amount of insulin down, is simply about hitting those targets. And I mean, getting under those daily targets. That's **120g** for those on *Wave*, **90g** for those on *Blaze*, and **60g** for those on *Quake*.

IF YOU WANT TO BE SKINNY, YOU MUST REAL-IZE THAT YOUR TOTAL DAILY CARB INTAKE IS

THE BIGGEST DIET FACTOR TO AFFECT YOUR SUCCESS. THAT'S WHY I'VE USED BOLD TYPE, CAPITALS, AND EVEN UNDERLINED IT! B.T.W ITALICS DIDN'T LOOK RIGHT!

I can't emphasize it much more than that! Up to this point, I actually avoided using all three font enhancements at the same time, just so *that* sentence could get maximum impact! Seriously, whatever you read outside of this book, that's *the* critical skinny factor!

Okay, I'll stop shouting now and using so many exclamation marks. I promise that if you keep your total daily carbs where they need to be, and use some or all of the other ideas in this book, you'll completely shock yourself within 6 weeks.

FINALLY, FOR THOSE WHO SPOTTED THE * EARLIER

There are 12 common vegetables that don't really deserve to be given 'eat-as-much-as-you-like' status. I'm not saying they're unhealthy. Not at all. And I'm not even saying that you can't eat them. But if you do eat them, do count their carbs.

Baked beans, Beetroot, Carrots, Parsnips, Peas, Plantain, Potatoes, Pumpkin, Squash, Sweet corn, Water chestnut, Yam

GET THE SKINNY ON...

OMG 6 You don't need carbs to survive

OMG 5 Higher carb diets stop you burning your body fat

OMG 4 Don't eat more than 4 iPhones or Blackberrys worth of pure carbs

OMG 3 Keep carbs at smart levels and you'll lose body fat faster

OMG 2 You'll also burn ketones, a fuel made from your body fat

OMG 1 You don't need to count the carbs in most vegetables

OMG ! Get under your daily carb limit and you'll burn fat fast!

THE TRUTH ABOUT BEING NAUGHTY

Now you know that to get skinny fast, you need to get your total daily carbs down to a smart level. And some of you might be asking, 'does it matter what type of carbs I eat?'. Here's your answer. Dietitians and doctors, I'd look away now.

In lucky people or those with willpower, *to get skinny*, it makes no difference whether they get all their daily carbs from cans of *Coke* or from plates of broccoli.

What's up doc? Read the sentence again and look out for the italics. I said, *to get skinny*, at least for some people, it makes no difference where they get their carbs from. I know, it's hard to believe. And no, I don't work for *Coca Cola!*

In terms of general health, of course it's smart to pick the best foods to live on. The body is built cell by cell, and if you use the best quality ingredients, you'll make the best quality finished product. If you use crap ingredients, well, you get it.

How could you get skinny by using poor quality carbs? As I said, you either have to be lucky or have willpower. If you find that's you, roll with it. Now for the second time today, doctors and dietitians, please cover your eyes.

In the past few years, people have been trying really hard to shift their fat. Many different theories have sprung up in the quest to find skinny perfection. And now we have the rise of the *research scientists*. Like us, they don't care about theory.

They care about results. Statistics. Facts. Pounds of fat lost. Pounds regained. They probably even dream in numbers! And I'm truly happy that they exist. Because recently, a few of the smartest geeks in town spotted something cool.

They analyzed hundreds of diets, and thousands of people. And although their discovery didn't hit the news, the boffins had found a needle in a haystack. In *some* of us, total daily carbs, not type of carbs, completely predicted fat loss.

It's the sort of news that no one wants to admit, because it risks undoing years of government campaigns to make us eat better. Smart scientists who live in our world, know that many people *just* care about being skinny!

Anyway, the news got squashed. So I've unsquashed it. In fact I just invented a new word at the same time! For a few weeks, definitely 6 and maybe 12, there's no harm in using this knowledge to get super skinny. I mean, make carb totals top priority.

It's much healthier to lose excess body fat fast, even if the methods used aren't ideal for a whole lifetime. **Every second that you're fat, you're damaging your health and your confidence. Screw tradition, and save both *right now*.**

Back to those *Coke* swillers. Their muscles deal with carbs well, as do most systems in their body. All they need to do is make sure that their daily carb totals are low. They still can't have any amount of carbs, but they can have any kind.

If you are able to do this, remember that while losing fat is a form of getting healthy, it's not the whole enchilada. Even if you don't care about long-term health, I bet you care about your skin and hair! Eventually they'll cry if you don't feed them well.

YOU PLUCKY GIRL

Some people don't find it easy to get skinny on poor quality carbs. But, they *still* manage it. And this is because they have super **willpower**. These plucky girls literally tell their body what to do, instead of the other way around.

When I say willpower, I mean the ability to control how much goes in your mouth. And that's the main problem if you don't have this mental strength. Poorer quality carbs can make it easy to overeat in general.

For someone with willpower, this is no problem. They stop eating when they decide to, and refuse to cave in to hunger. Very few have this toughness to defeat 2,000,000 years of genetic design! But they do exist. And it could be you.

If you're lucky or plucky, you can still get skinny by eating the worst junk carbs on the planet, as long as you don't have too many. This isn't ideal for your whole life, but if it helps you beat daily carb targets for 6 to 12 weeks, do it.

What would this mean in the real world? Maybe that some could have a chicken breast and a naughty *Coke* for lunch, and still lose fat. As long as daily carb totals weren't exceeded, it wouldn't matter where those carbs came from.

I can already hear some of you figuring how much chocolate it would take to fill your entire daily carb totals! This section isn't meant to make you choose the worst quality carbs. It's a reminder to **keep those carb totals down at all costs**.

WHO AM I?

How would you know if you're like this? The only way to find out is by doing. If you always manage to beat the daily carb totals, good for you, keep it up. And if you're struggling, or want better general health, you might like the next chapter.

GET THE SKINNY ON...

OMG 6 Keeping total daily carbs down is ultra important

OMG 5 For some people just doing that can make them skinny

OMG 4 Ignoring carb quality can be okay for 6 to 12 weeks

OMG 3 Once you get skinny, start to look at carb quality

OMG 2 Carb quality affects long-term general health in all of us

OMG 1 Poor quality carbs make it easy to overeat in some people

OMG ! If getting your carbs down is tough, read the next chapter!

THE FAST AND THE FURIOUS: PART 1

Way back at the start, I said that I believed in helping you understand stuff, instead of getting you to just *do what I say.* I still believe that. So, for those of you who don't feel lucky or plucky, here's the 101 on picking better quality carbs.

Some carbs are fast and furious. Some are just fast, and others are just furious. The best are neither. And at this point you're thinking, 'what's this all about?'. This section might be repetitive (like the entire book!) but stick it out.

What do I mean by 'fast'? I mean the speed at which you can get a carb from your plate to your stomach. When carbs make this journey too rapidly, you're setting up a big problem. And yes, I did mean the pun! What is this big problem?

You'll eat too many carbs overall. In terms of this book, it means you'll always go over the daily carb totals. And in terms of life, you'll always struggle to keep skinny. Old genes can't cope with modern food speeding down the throat freeway!

Too many carbs reaching the stomach at once causes alarm bells to ring. Too much 'food traffic' means that your body must release lots of insulin. Too much insulin means that your body must convert some of this carb traffic jam into body fat.

Fast carbs are carbs which travel from your plate to your stomach too easily. They make it extremely difficult to keep under your daily carb limits.

LEAVING OUT LEPTIN

Another reason that fast carbs cause a problem, is because you consume too many before leptin gets a chance to warn you. If you've forgotten, leptin is like your body's gas gauge. It tells you when you've had enough fuel (food).

To help leptin work, eating meals instead of snacks is a good start. The next thing is to not eat too fast. Although it's hard to measure, there does seem to be around a 20 minute delay for your brain to compute how much food you've eaten.

Carbs make up a big chunk of modern food, and can often sneak past leptin and stop it doing its job. Leptin is there to help us. By preventing you eating too much, it keeps your insulin down, which allows you to get back to burning body fat sooner.

Simply by eating carbs that travel from plate to stomach quickly, you're preventing leptin, your body's fuel gauge, from telling you when to stop eating. Avoid fast carbs for this reason alone. Or eat in slow motion!

LIQUID LUNCH

So, who are these fast travelling carbs? **The first baddies are liquid carbs**. I haven't forgotten about just mentioning *Coke*. Some don't need this info, some do. In nature, ready-to-drink liquid carbs are rare. There's breast, cow and coconut milk. And honey. Beyond that, there's not much!

Now look in your local grocery store. I expect you'll see a whole wall of liquid carbs. When you have any liquid, even ones that start as something natural, like a fruit smoothie, it becomes easy for some people to overdo carbs.

Let's take the example of a smoothie further, and say it's made from four fruits. A banana, orange, pineapple and some strawberries. If you were to mix those in nature, it would take you weeks. For a start, you'd have to find them!

Bananas don't grow near strawberries. Let's be kind and say that they do. You'd still take time and effort to mix them up into a modern shake. Individually, fruits (with meals) are okay. But once they become liquids, they become the opposite.

Liquid carbs also speed because they slip down your throat. This is how seagulls eat fish (note to self: *I don't have wings*). Solid or semi-solid foods travel through your digestive system in a much slower, pulse-like process called peristalsis.

If you have a tough time getting your carb totals down, the easiest first step is to avoid all liquid carbs. It might take some mental adjustment, especially if you're used to drinking liquid carbs with meals. Hey, I find water boring too!

MAXIMUM MUNCH

What else can make carbs speed demons? I call it maximum munch. Sounds silly, but the point behind it isn't. By maximum munch, I mean how much of a food you can get physically get into your mouth at any one moment.

I realize that you might be viewing this as non-scientific. Let me give you some real life examples. Okay, which is easier to eat: potatoes or French fries? Corn or popcorn? Brown rice or white rice? It's not a trick question.

The correct answers are French fries, popcorn and white rice! But not for the obvious reasons you might think. Apart from being a liquid, many factors affect maximum munch. Let's take a look at the most important.

THE FIBER TRAFFIC COP

If a food has lots of fiber, it's physically tougher to eat than food with less. It will require more chews than gulps. Many foods, and I don't just mean liquids, only need gulps! And for some people, that's just too much of a temptation.

Fiber is the part of a food we can't digest, made from a plant's cell walls. Scientists give props to fiber as something that 'fills you up'. True, but yet again, they've not seen the obvious. High-fiber foods make a difference *before* they reach your stomach.

Brown rice has more fiber than white, making it chewy and harder to eat. Fiber also swells with water and saliva, making it even slower to chow down. So, high-fiber foods give you stuff to do (chew!), which often makes you eat less of them.

What's a high or low fiber food? You could go for numbers, and say anything with more than 3 grams per serving is 'high'.

A simpler option is just to **pick the higher fiber version whenever you see two similar foods side by side**.

SOFTLY SOFTLY QUICKLY

Let's go back to the potatoes and French fries. Now I'm not talking about calories, just the carbs. The French fries make it extremely easy to get carbs from mouth to stomach fast. Why? Because they've been softened.

Cooking, chopping, mashing or processing, e.g. turning sugar canes into sugar grains. Lots of stuff softens food. It's not important how it happens. What's important is **softer carbs are easy to overeat and blitz your stomach**.

Here's another simple test. Ask yourself, 'would this food dissolve or crumble in my mouth?'. If the answer is 'yes', find something better. Rice cakes, a food adored by many dieters, fails this test too easily! As for cookies...

THE AWKWARD CUSTOMER

Many foods are awkward to eat. And that's great! Although you'd never eat sweet corn in the movies, it's worth making a comparison with cousin popcorn. The corn on the cob version is much slower to eat than the one you can claw at!

And actually, in nature, almost all foods are awkward to get from your hand to your stomach fast. It's like Mother Nature knew that if she made something quick to eat, we'd simply eat more of it! So, she can be a smart mom.

So there you have fast carbs. Foods which travel from mouth to stomach in a flash. The faster a carb makes this journey, the more you'll overeat them. Pretty basic, but basics are always looked over. Liquids are the worst. Also watch out for low-fiber, super soft and easy-grab carbs too.

GET THE SKINNY ON...

OMG 6 Fast carbs travel from plate to stomach too quickly

OMG 5 This makes them much easier to overeat

OMG 4 You might go over your daily carb totals too easily

OMG 3 This raises insulin which stops you burning body fat

OMG 2 Fast carbs stop leptin from switching off your appetite

OMG 1 Liquids, low-fiber and soft foods are typical fast carbs

OMG ! Choose fiddly, solid and high-fiber carbs more often!

THE FAST AND THE FURIOUS:
PART 2

Some carbs are furious. Does that mean they're angry? No. But they certainly make your body angry. And eventually, if you keep flinging them down the calorie chute, they'll make *you* furious when you look in the mirror!

Furious describes a carb's ability to aggressively raise your blood sugar level. After total daily carbs, it's the next biggest factor to affect your chance of achieving skinny success.

PANIC ATTACKS

If carbs get digested fast, they're turning into glucose, *fast*. And when all that glucose hits the bloodstream, the body panics. This is because **too much glucose in the blood is dangerous and damages cells**. Of course, the body has an emergency plan.

It releases insulin. This grabs hold of the excess glucose, and *dumps* it. It dumps some in muscles, who store and use it when necessary. And it dumps lots inside fat cells, who gleefully turn it *into* more body fat. **This is how most humans get fat**.

In an ideal world, your body would produce a dinky drop of insulin and top-up your muscles with glucose. Your fat cells would be left moaning, 'hey, what about us?'. The insulin would rise after a meal, and settle down smoothly.

HOW TO RUIN A PARTY

It's time to remember something important. **You can only burn body fat if there's no insulin hanging around**. Insulin is like a bad party guest. You know they're coming over, so you just want them in and out as soon as possible!

Problem is, some guests don't know when they're not wanted. Once they're through the door (you eat), they linger around! This means that you spend less time partying (burning body fat) and more time waiting for the clown to leave!

It's a lose-lose scenario, and something you must avoid. The best sources of carbs won't do this. The worst will ruin your party. So, let's delve deeper and see exactly who deserves to make your guest list.

DRINKING GAMES

Straight off, don't invite any liquids over! As I mentioned in the fast section, liquids travel way too quickly. Liquids are a bunch of jocks that rock-up all at once. And when they arrive at your home (your stomach), watch out!

Liquid carbs eliminate your stomach's first job, to turn solid into liquid. Liquid's head start means that it converts to glucose with frightening speed. When you *flood the blood* like this, your body must release a surge of insulin.

Dangerous liquids are the same as all furious carbs. They're like a rocket, shooting your blood sugar high and fast. This truly is the 'sugar rush'. Liquid carbs are like a successful hunting trip in a bottle. Not natural at all.

PLEASE SIR, CAN I HAVE SOME MORE?

When blood sugar skyrockets, a chemical called **dopamine** does the same. This feel-good chemical is a reward. The brain thinks you've found a banana tree and climbed 30 foot to get one (while naked)! Dopamine memorizes 'yay' moments.

The more intense the dopamine release, the more you'll become 'obsessed' at getting the feeling again. **This is how carb addiction starts**. Furious carbs drive you to find MORE, day after day. You might even climb trees naked!

Because you've reached new heights of dopamine excitement, everything after seems a bit *boring*. You can see how furious carbs soon redefine what food you crave. It's not easy, but with time you can learn how to train your dragon.

Furious carbs raise your blood sugar fast and high. Your brain notices this and release dopamine, a feel-good chemical. This memorizes 'the rush' and makes you seek it out again and again. Furious carbs make you really miss food.

Even after all the excess carbs have been cleared away, there's still some insulin floating around. Why? Because the body panicked and made too much in the first place. And **with insulin in the blood, you can't burn any body fat**.

These high levels of insulin have been known to stay elevated for 9 hours after a large pizza. Talk about a massive 'slice' of your fat burning day ruined! Less furious carbs will drop insulin back down after 2 to 3 hours.

Furious carbs raise blood sugar fast, and to cope, your body pumps out insulin. In a panic, it releases too much. This forces floating carbs into fat cells, converting them *into* body fat. Insulin stays up even after all the excess sugar is gone. **If there's insulin in your blood, you can't burn body fat**. I'm being repetitive for a reason.

Let's get back to what makes carbs furious guests who ruin the fat burning party. Once you can picture the usual suspects, you won't be so confused about food any more. Instead, you'll develop an instinct for picking the best carbs.

FIBER (AGAIN!)

You've already learned that fiber slows down the speed that you can eat something. It also slows down digestion *in* the stomach. This stops your body converting carbs into glucose so quickly. And that helps *stop* you making a panic-sized portion of insulin (i.e. a supersized amount).

Soluble fiber does it best. In your stomach, it turns gloopy and makes a meal tougher to mash up. That means a trickle of carbs enter your blood. At that speed, your brain gets a drink, and muscles can use the rest. Insulin sits pretty (low).

The best sources of soluble fiber are plants with tough skin. Skin is where the fiber's at. Apples have lots, oats too. You don't need to seek out fiber, but if you have a choice, a higher fiber carb choice serves you best.

SILLY SUPPLEMENTS

There is also a supplement called *psyllium* (sounds like 'silly - ahem'). This is fiber made from tiny seeds on the skin of a plantain (a cousin of the fruit you climb trees naked for). A similar product is called *guar gum*. Be careful with these.

I mention them simply because I know that many readers will seek out everything possible to help them lose fat. These fiber supplements are popular with dieters. Although they're generally safe (especially psyllium), they have risks.

Soluble fiber literally means that it dissolves in water. Imagine it as a sponge. If you don't have enough water, it will soak up everything you have in your digestive system, and create a blockage. Drink lots of water if you use them.

GOLD, SILVER AND BRONZE SUGARS

Okay, this is the crucial one. Follow this and you'll be well on your way to avoiding a furious response. When we first met carbs, I explained that they were made from different numbers of 'bits'. The bits being *types* of sugars.

Generally, problem carbs are those made from one or two bits. They're too easy to split. When carbs *snap* easy, they convert into glucose, easy. That raises insulin easy, yada yada yada, you get the drill now. **You get fat easy!**

Modern foods have lots of these sugars added to them. They're everywhere. Food companies know how addictive sugar is. You could call modern food companies the inventors of dopamine! Sugar addiction equals *kerching*.

The problem with sugar is mainly when we *add* it to foods. The only added sugar that's slightly safe, is the sugar added by nature in the first place! The most furious carb foods always have sugar added by man. Or by woman. Pets are innocent.

I have a golden rule about avoiding the furious sugars. Actually, it's a golden, silver and bronze rule. Food labels list ingredients in size order, heaviest first. Vitamins, minerals and flavors are last, because they're light in weight.

If you see 'sugar' in gold, silver or bronze medal positions, that's 1st, 2nd or 3rd place, you need to be honest. Eating that means you're mainly eating sugar, with just a hint of the food you actually wanted!

Any gold, silver or bronze sugar will make your body furious. Either the food part tastes bad without it, or the company just wants to make an addict out of you. Either way, say sayonara! It would be better labeled, 'Sugar. Also contains some food'!

It's not always easy to spot this furious fiend. Why? Companies are getting careful and hiding the 's' word. There are now so many types of sugar, that listing foods with them would be impossible. But we have a three letter savior (not *that* one!).

WATCH OUT FOR TH O – S – E

These little babies are a big clue if you want to avoid furious carbs. I won't attempt to make a clever anagram from

them! Whenever you see '…ose' at the end of an ingredient, it's sugar, and it has been *added*. **One hundred percent furious.**

Want me to name a few? 'Sucrose', 'fructose', 'lactose', 'dextrose', 'maltose', 'high-fructose corn syrup (HFCS)', 'glucose syrup', 'polydextrose'. The list goes on. **Just look for the letters, 'ose'.**

There are newer, even sneakier versions of added sugar now. They include, 'beet sugar', 'cane juice', 'barley malt', 'turbinado sugar' and 'dextrin'. If you're unsure, buy it, eat it, and *Google* the suspect for next time! **Only you can protect yourself.**

If aliens visited us, they'd be confused by the efforts we make to grow amazing food, and then mix all of them with one common ingredient, sugar. They'd surely assume that it was a powerful drug which kept our species alive!

The easy way to avoid furious carbs, is to watch out for foods with added sugar in the first 3 ingredients. You'll usually see the word sugar, or something ending in the letters 'ose'. Find and flush these out, and you'll get skinny *much* **faster.**

If you avoid those major league fury factors, you'll get skinny quickly. Avoid liquid carbs, don't eat anything with sugar or 'ose' in the first 3 ingredients, and pick higher fiber carbs when you have a choice. Anything else?

THE MINOR LEAGUE

There are many other factors that affect how furious a carb will be. To be straight with you, they make a difference, but it's usually small. And also, they're things that you might find difficult to control. Still, for those who want to know it all...

HOT TEMPERED

The more you cook certain foods, the more furious they get. And it's not literally because you're eating them hot! Once cooked foods have cooled down (or even if you freeze them), they'll still be more furious than if they were never cooked. Why?

Cooking breaks apart the structure of food. Especially carbs, which tend to be weaker than protein or fat. Breaking up the structure is simply like starting the digestion process before you've even touched the food.

Take pasta. It's slightly furious. But go authentic and undercook it *al dente* style (Italian for *to the bite*), and it will be tougher to digest, and less furious to the body. Personally, I prefer un-authentic, and *love* my penne soft! As I said, minor league factors.

So, foods which are cooked the least will be the toughest to digest, and the least furious. What are these foods? Anything less cooked! You don't have to eat raw food always. It's just nice knowing that if you can't start camp fires, you'll survive and even thrive!

RIPE FOR THE PICKING

If you eat fruit or vegetables when they're fresh, they'll be less furious than if you wait around and eat them 3 days later. A yellow banana with hints of green is much less furious than a yellow banana with leopard spots.

This is because fruit and vegetables have chemicals which gradually break down their own sugar content (fruits have the most sugar). In fact, we've discovered that picking fruit starts this ripening process. It starts them digesting themselves. Nice.

Breaking down their own sugar means that we don't have to do it as much. So, ripe fruits and vegetables react more furiously in the body. It's difficult to measure, but worth knowing. Eating fresh makes sense if you can.

And that's a mighty chapter for you to digest. It might make you want to put the book down fast, or just *be* furious! Understanding stuff is important. Otherwise you'll be stuck reading diet books for life, instead of living it.

GET THE SKINNY ON...

OMG 6 Furious carbs cause massive panic once inside you

OMG 5 They force insulin to skyrocket high and long

OMG 4 This stops you burning your body fat for ages

OMG 3 Furious carbs boost dopamine which makes food addictive

OMG 2 Liquid carbs, low-fiber carbs and overcooked carbs are furious

OMG 1 Man-made sugars are the commonest furious carbs in our diet

OMG ! Steer clear of foods which have '…ose' in the first 3 ingredients!

SWEET AND DEADLY

We think about fruit as something that's healthy. And almost no expert or member of the public would disagree. Fruit has vitamins, minerals, fiber, undiscovered phyto chemicals (plant chemicals), and it tastes good!

But is that it, is fruit an angel? Not really. Because if you're trying to shift the fat, fruit can be a cheeky devil! Its legendary levels of anti-oxidants (chemicals that stop us oxidizing, which means rusting, which means ageing!) and its naturalness are without question.

Don't get seduced by this smooth talking *nature is nice* vibe. Hailstones are part of nature too! Fruit, depending on which kind, can have quite high levels of a sugar called **fructose**, neatly known as **fruit sugar**. And **fructose can cause chaos**.

FRUIT INCREASES YOUR APPETITE

That seems like a strange statement. Especially if you have a memory of having a piece of fruit, and it making you satisfied for a bit. But overall, fruit, if it's one with high levels of fructose, causes your appetite to get out of whack.

It doesn't *directly* increase appetite, but it stops our friend leptin from doing its job. If you've forgotten, leptin is the fuel gauge which tells us when to stop eating. Fruit containing lots of fructose, *stops* leptin from doing this.

Even if you eat meals, which are normally good at boosting leptin, fructose blocks it from telling our brain that we've eaten enough. It's almost like fructose wraps its hand around leptin's mouth, and stops it from speaking up. Cheeky parrot!

FRUIT CALORIES SLIP UNDER YOUR RADAR

Most calories raise leptin. The more you have, the more leptin increases, and the quicker your appetite shuts off. That's how it's *supposed* to work. But **fruit doesn't raise leptin at all**. Fruit's supposed to be a health food not a stealth food!

So, if you have fruit with food, it adds calories to the total, but the leptin can't *see* them. If the calories weren't from fructose, leptin might be able to work out that you'd eaten enough. But it doesn't do this with fruit.

This double whammy of adding secret calories and stopping the leptin controlling our appetite, is dangerous. Don't even get me started on the concept of fruits being 'perfect for snacking'! But there's more.

FRUIT STOPS INSULIN WORKING

Fruit's sugar, fructose, gives insulin a hard time. Remember, it's insulin that takes the carbs out of the blood and puts them in muscle or fat cells. Fructose stop muscles and our liver from absorbing excess carbs. So where do these calories go?

Fat cells. They're a motel with a neon sign that always says, 'VACANCY'! Fructose stops muscles from being their normal sponge-like self, and lets fat cells lock up the calories instead. Sneaky. Some **proof that nature intended fruit to be a treat**.

Our liver, which is where fruit's fructose is broken down, can only get through about 200 calories of the stuff per day, especially when dieting. That's not a huge amount. I'm not saying that you have to avoid fruit completely, just be careful.

What is careful? The smart thing is to choose fruits that are lower in fructose. Fruit juices are worse than solid fruit, because you can easily *drink* more fructose than you can *eat*, which means more calories going *unnoticed*.

The new trend of home blender drinks, and ready-made versions sold in store's chilled areas, are keeping huge waddling crowds of health-conscious people, *fat*. **They might be full of nutrients, but there's no such thing as an innocent smoothie!**

I suggest different amounts of fruit depending on what plan level you're on, and only with meals. Check out the section on **crop rotation** and use various fruits to get a variety of healthy nutrients over the 6 weeks and beyond. **You don't** *have* **to eat fruit**.

To be fair, fruit isn't the only source of fructose. In fact, wherever you see fructose, it's best to be aware of the facts. Fruit gets a special mention, mainly because it has a rep of untouchable goodness, which just isn't accurate.

HIGH FRUCTOSE CORN SYRUP

While we're here, it's a logical time to mention this. Although no food eaten once is immediately bad, there are some things which border on the ridiculous. **High Fructose Corn Syrup** is ridiculous. This stuff makes fruit seem like an angel again!

It's a syrup made from corn (obviously!), and over *half* of its calories are from fructose. Also known as **Glucose Fructose Syrup**, it's used now in a massive variety of foods, including soups, yogurts, breads, cereals and breakfast bars. Even 'health' foods.

But the big place where it ends up (apart from your butt!), is in soft drinks, like colas, lemonades and energy formulas. It adds *extreme sweetness*, and as you might already guess, it causes absolute *chaos* inside.

Its calories go undetected, it stops other calories from being talked about (i.e. it blocks the brain from hearing that you're full), and it makes muscles poor at absorbing the excess carbs. If you want to lose fat fast, avoid it when you can.

Yes, there *are* people who won't notice *any* difference if they eat fruits or not, or *even* have lots of high fructose corn syrup. But you need to have lucky genes or be mentally tough to avoid overeating if you make best friends with fructose.

Whoever you are, it will probably be easier if you stick to the advices here, or at least see fruit in an accurate light. Like many things, the only way to truly find out how a food affects you, is to try it, and keep an eye on it.

FRUIT BOWL RECOMMENDATIONS

WAVE - up to 3 fruits per day (one in each meal but ideally *avoid* it in meal 3)

BLAZE - up to 2 fruits per day (one in meals 1 and 2)

QUAKE - up to 1 fruit per day (one in meal 1)

Eat fruit at the end of a meal so that leptin has a chance to work out how many calories you've already stocked up on. And if possible, avoid fruit in meal 3 to reduce the chance of breaking your fuel gauge (leptin) so close to sleep.

LOW-FRUCTOSE FRUITS (PICK THESE)

Avocados, blueberries, grapefruits, guava, lemons, limes, pineapple, plums, strawberries and tomato (it is a fruit!)

HIGH-FRUCTOSE FRUITS (DON'T HAVE THESE TOO OFTEN)

All dried fruits including apricots, dates, figs, mango, papaya, peaches, pears, prunes, raisins, *Zante* currants (also known as currants!).

MEDIUM-FRUCTOSE FRUITS (PICK THESE ONCE YOU'VE GOT YOUR IDEAL BODY)

Any fruit which isn't mentioned in the first two categories, is probably in this one. During your 6 weeks, try and pick from the first list (if you can call it a list!) and some from 'here'. Avoid the others until you're super skinny.

GET THE SKINNY ON . . .

OMG 6 Fruit is healthy because it contains fiber and many nutrients

OMG 5 Fruit also contains a simple sugar called fructose

OMG 4 Fructose stops leptin from helping us control our appetite

OMG 3 Fructose makes muscles bad at absorbing excess carbs

OMG 2 If carbs get swallowed up by fat cells you will get heavier

OMG 1 Pick lower fructose fruits when you can

OMG ! Have up to 3 pieces of fruit per day and only with meals!

CARBS IN A NUTSHELL

Hold on, nuts don't have carbs! Too late, I've written it now. This is a quick chapter to sum up everything you've learnt or not learnt about carbs. A book editor would say this chapter is repetitive and not needed. And guess what, they'd be a fat blimp of an editor!

1. DON'T HAVE TOO MANY CARBS

At least get this. Carbs produce insulin, and insulin stops you burning body fat. Done. Keep carbs down to these amounts for 6 weeks. Don't count the carbs in vegetables. Get under these daily totals whenever you can:

WAVE - Have up to **120** grams per day

BLAZE - Have up to **90** grams per day

QUAKE - Have up to **60** grams per day

If you're stuck and can't be sure how many carbs are in your food, think 'phone'. That's 2 *iPhones* or *Blackberrys* next to each other, and 2 more on top of them. It's an emergency guide. Don't eat more. And don't eat the phones. It's harder to text.

2. AVOID THE FAST AND FURIOUS

Fast carbs are easy to eat carbs. They'll push you over your daily target. Furious carbs raise your blood sugar super high.

They rocket insulin, which blocks fat loss for hours. They also boost dopamine, which makes you a carb addict.

Liquid carbs are fast and furious. Pour them away! Low fiber carbs are easy to eat and digest. Avoid them. Foods with sugar in the first 3 ingredients aren't even foods! Avoid them. If you see 'ose' in the ingredients, put it down!

Good job! There's always other stuff, but **if you manage to understand and apply the above carb basics, you'll be a long way towards living in Skinnyville**. And guess what, if you've forgotten already...

GET THE SKINNY ON...

OMG 6 Zero carb diets are rubbish and so are regular carb diets

OMG 5 Keeping carbs low lets you burn body fat throughout the day

OMG 4 Avoid fast carbs which make it easier to exceed daily carb totals

OMG 3 Avoid furious carbs that block fat loss and addict you to food

OMG 2 As a rough guide don't eat more than 4 iPhones or Blackberrys

OMG 1 You don't need to count the carbs in your vegetables

OMG ! Start by seeing if you can get under 120 grams of carbs in total!

BIG FAT LIES

We're obsessed with the word 'low'. Low prices, low stress and low energy are just three of the lows that excite us. And then there's the 'low' that seems to beat all the others, **low-fat**. For such a small phrase, it gets such a big reaction when we see it!

But are we right to be excited about this particular low? No! So, why does seeing 'low-fat' make us happy? Because we've been tricked! Food companies who want to make big money use two things: smart marketing and dumb science. How?

For most of human history, we didn't hate or avoid dietary fat. We just viewed it as a part of food, and left it at that. And for *all* that time, most humans were definitely skinny. Dietary fat was just another cool kid at school. Fat was phat!

People weren't skinny just because 'they were more physical back then'. Studies show that there wasn't much of a difference compared to today. And if you visit a modern gym, *trust me*, you'll see lots of very energetic people, who are still very fat!

But something happened in the 1960s. Too many people started dying from heart attacks. The scientists investigated. Pretty soon they decided that they'd solved the problem: we were eating too much fat. And the solution? Fire a silver bullet: cut out fat in the diet.

But **they were wrong**. After World War 2 ended, there were lots of chemicals lying around, chemicals normally used for making bombs and other explosives. As economies were in ruin, people didn't want to waste anything.

So, the chemicals found their way into the hands of farmers, who noticed that if they added them to soil, crops would grow faster and stronger. This, my smart friend, was **the birth of fertilizer**. And baby, did we fertilize fields and fields of carbs!

With the war done and everyone in party mode, we ate more food than ever before. At the same time, food's spiritual partner turned up. Color TV arrived! And with TV came the commercials to sell us stuff. Guess what we bought? It has 5 letters and starts with 'c'.

We bought bread, cereals, soft drinks, cookies, cakes, 'TV dinners', and even foods that most of us had never eaten before (like rice and exotic fruits). The amount of carbs in our diets skyrocketed, and they've never come back down!

Carbs were made to look sexy, good for you, exciting and fresh. Some of the most famous food commercials in history were made during this time. Slowly and secretly, people were getting fat from the carbs, and that *did* increase heart disease.

Looking back, you could say that the scientists were just doing what was logical, and were under pressure to find a bad guy. Maybe. But in reality, the protein and carb industries had people protecting them. **Fat had no friends**.

So, with no one to stand by them, poor old fat was turned into a nasty villain. Even today, fat is still serving time for a crime it

135

didn't commit! And that's unfair, with lots of modern research finding proof that fat was innocent all along.

With science suggesting we *'should* cut fat down', and with TV commercials pushing carbs, the obvious thing happened. **Low-fat arrived**. But how do companies actually make a 'low-fat' product? Surely they just cut the fat out?

That would be logical. But they can't *just* cut the fat out. If you kept cutting things out of food packages, they'd become tiny! You could add some water back. That helps keep it big and heavy, but too much water tends to dilute flavor.

What have they got left? You could add protein. The trouble is, protein is expensive, it doesn't last long on the shelf, and it actually *stops* customers from overeating. No profit-making company wants that to happen!

One thing left. Take out the fat, and replace it with carbs. Carbs are cheap to grow (blame World War 2's accidental fertilizer discovery), they last for ages on the shelf, and here's the real beauty: they're very, very, addictive.

CARB DEALER

Carbs are the diamonds of nature's food. And I don't mean they're a girl's best friend! I mean, they're rare. Being such a rare treat, when we eat them, they trigger a chemical in the brain that makes us feel good. Dopamine. Why *hello*, we've met already.

This is the closest we get to Mother Nature being naughty. Around the globe, she scattered tiny amounts of very addictive drug-like substances. And we call these drugs, *carbs*. Boy oh boy did carbs sneak past the 'don't do drugs' campaign!

In small amounts, at the right time, carbs are okay. Unfortunately, because we've got so good at making them on a huge scale, we've become victims of them. We are the carb addicts and food companies are the carb dealers!

Look at me, I've forgotten about our old friend, fat. Even though it can look greasy, feel slimy and taste fatty, fat isn't a villain. **If you eat a lower carb diet, fat from your plate is mostly used for energy.** I mean that. Scout's honor.

If you become obsessed about avoiding fat in your food, you'll automatically pick foods that are high in carbs. High carbs *will* make you fat. Almost all modern foods that are marketed as 'low-fat', will be very high in carbs.

Starting *today*, get the 'low-fat' idea out of your head. The worst products tend to be those advertised as '99% fat free' or similar. When you see *such* high percentages, it means that they *must* have a high percentage of something else. You got it!

In fact, some of those '99% fat-free' foods are close to 99% carbs! And that's an incredible 'achievement' of modern science. In nature, those kinds of figures hardly exist. **The majority of our low-fat foods are simply not natural.**

PETER PAN: THE REAL VILLAIN

There's one type of fat that *is* evil. It doesn't occur in nature, but it does occur in stores. It's called **trans fat** (just think of *Dracula's* home, *Transylvania*). Also known as **hydrogenated fat**, you can find it lurking in baked goods like chips and cookies.

Before it was invented, we used to make cookies and similar foods with butter, or other animal fats. The problem was, they didn't keep fresh. After a few weeks on the shelf, natural fats tend to react with air and become disgusting.

So, thanks to some pesky scientists, we got an evil 'solution'. They found that by squeezing vegetable seeds for their oil, and firing hydrogen atoms at it, they could create a modern fat that never gets old. *Peter Pan* fats!

These fats cause problems with our heart, probably make insulin go wrong, and may even increase some cancers. The WHO (the who? The World Health Organization!) recommend that we have a maximum of 1% of our calories from them.

In other words, *don't* have them. The 1% is the WHO realizing that these fats are lurking everywhere, and getting rid of them completely is unlikely. I've seen the research, and I recommend this: **totally avoid trans / hydrogenated fats if you spot them**.

They're listed on labels in most countries, and if you see them, *run*. They have no benefit to the human body, and there will always be an alternative version of the food you want that *doesn't* contain them. Avoid *Peter Pan* immediately!

THE PHAT FATS!

Fats have had a rough ride this section. We've seen that they've been accused of a crime they didn't commit, and have been in jail since the 1960s. And we've seen that the real villains, carbs, are allowed to walk the streets (our throats) freely.

We've discovered that if you're generally on a lower carb diet, dietary fat will simply be used for energy. And finally, we've seen that there's one fat, the *Peter Pan* fat, which never ages, which is toxic and which must be killed off.

There's one final bit of the fat story. The fat good guys! These are two fat brothers that are important for our health, and they can actually help us *lose* body fat. These fats are so useful, you could even call them *essential*. And that's them.

THE DON'T LEAVE HOME WITHOUT THEM, FATS

They're actually called **essential fats**. Mainly because if you don't ever have them, you'll die. But why? Our brain, which is mainly fat, is particularly made from these. And so are the walls of millions of our cells. No brain, no cells? It's a no brainer!

These fats also reduce inflammation in the body, they help eyesight develop properly, and they might even boost intelligence. I see you nodding your head at all that, and secretly wanting to shout, 'yeah, nice, but will they make me look good?'!

THE FAT SENSITIVE GUY

Yes. They do two cool things. Firstly, they make sure that insulin works properly. And they do this by making your muscle cells work well *with* insulin, so that they absorb any excess carbs in the blood.

This is **improving insulin sensitivity**. Picture this. If carbs show up to muscle's door, and it's rude (i.e. not sensitive), the carbs will be upset and go visit your body fat's doors. And *they'll* be all nice and say, 'why there's always more room at the *Fat-Inn*, please come in'!

If you keep putting carbs into your fat cells and let them get their wicked way, you'll get fat, fast. You ideally need any left over carbs to float around and *into* muscles, where they'll get stored temporarily until they're used. **Essential fats make muscles appealing**. Eat 'em.

THE FAT MESSENGER GUY

There's a second way that essential fats can help, and it's with appetite. Remember leptin? It's the chemical that tells you when you're full up. Well, essential fats make sure that leptin can get into the brain. Essential fats escort leptin to work each day.

People on high-carb diets tend to have low levels of essential fat. And because of this, their leptin (the main thing that tells them to stop eating) doesn't work. You can see that essential fats are essential if you want to get OMGs.

It's smart to get essential fats as often as you can. This can be tricky, as they're not commonly found in our food supply. You *can* find them in fish, and in some vegetable oils (supplements too). Females are good at using either of these sources.

The two fats are called **omega 3** and **omega 6**. You only need small amounts of them. I'm talking an amount that would fit on a spoon. If you eat fish twice per week, that will work. Fattier fish like salmon and trout have mega omegas in them.

If you hate fish, or love them enough to not kill them, you can get essential fats from vegetable oils. **Flax** oil (also called **linseed**) has decent amounts. And if you can't swallow slippery oil, you can get capsules from a health store (fish or vegetarian types).

These omega fats are really worth it. They have special benefits that we're only *just* discovering. If you're not convinced by these ideas, maybe give them a chance over these 6 weeks.

If you eat essential fats from food, i.e. fish, these can act as a source of protein too. One reason that fish is generally a good food, is because it contains those two nutrients, essential fat and essential protein, and nothing much else.

FOOD SOURCES OF ESSENTIAL FATS (HAVE ABOUT
TWICE PER WEEK)

Salmon

Mackerel

Trout

Sardines

Tuna

OIL SOURCES OF ESSENTIAL FATS
(HAVE ABOUT TWICE PER DAY)

Flax oil (a spoonful)

OTHER SOURCES OF ESSENTIAL FATS
(HAVE ONCE PER DAY)

Fish Oil capsules:

1 to 2 grams of fish oil per day

Don't have more than 2 grams per day, as it may weaken your immune system, making you sick. And if you're sick, you'll get sympathy food, you'll get bored, and you'll get fat!

Vegetarian capsules from *Algae* (it's just seaweed!):

DHA – 200mg or more, once per day

EPA – 100mg or more, once per day

(DHA and EPA are usually found together, so just get roughly these amounts)

I hope by now you're a bit more of a friend towards dietary fat. Don't be scared of it, and don't obsess about it. **Never count the calories or percent of fat**. If it's in a natural food, and if you're not eating high carbs, fat will be used for energy. Trust me.

And I hope you're super cautious of 'low-fat' foods. Realize that they're usually chock full of carbs, and are likely to be totally unnatural. This chapter takes a lot of faith to believe in. Give it a chance, and see the results for yourself.

GET THE SKINNY ON...

OMG 6 Eating dietary fat will not make you fat

OMG 5 Years ago people ate more dietary fat and were still way skinnier

OMG 4 Fat only has a bad rep due to scientific mistakes in the 1960s

OMG 3 Find essential fats (in fish, supplements or oils) and have them often

OMG 2 Avoid the Peter Pan fats completely (trans or hydrogenated)

OMG 1 Low-fat foods are pointless and have way too many fattening carbs

OMG ! Stop obsessing over dietary fat immediately!

HUNT AND WAIT

If you're female, you're not a hunter. In prehistory, the men were the hunters. All big and macho. The women made the cave look nice, and of course cooked for the guys when they came back after a long day's hunting. Right?

Would you really have waited patiently in a dark and damp cave all day, even 100,000 years ago? NO! My guess, and it's as good as the next cave dweller, is that you would have been out there, moving and doing *something*.

Your body doesn't care if you wear lipstick or not, it just cares that you're moving! Fat isn't a female thing. Fat is a human thing. Actually, fat is a *modern* human thing! Ancient humans just wouldn't be living like we do.

Earlier on, we talked about how important it was to get moving *first thing* in the morning. Making muscles work after a long gap (sleep), really melts the fat away. That first period of movement, **pom 1**, is *crucial*. But there's more.

HUNT, HUNT AND HUNT AGAIN

If you're eating three times per day, there are two more gaps between meals. There's one before your second meal, and one before your final munch. You may remember that **it's during**

long gaps that the body turns to burning body fat. So, can we use this couple of gaps?

Definitely! In fact, it would be unnatural if we didn't. Now, there would be no point if you moved around *just* after eating. When food arrives, your body won't allow fat burning. It just doesn't see the point, and besides, it ruins digestion.

But *a few hours after* you've eaten, your blood sugar would have dropped right down. **At this point, your body is ripe for more movement**. This burns some body fat right away, but even that's not as important compared to another benefit.

TELLING CARBS WHERE TO GO

When we eat carbs, they get turned into glucose. This floats around the blood, waiting for takers. Your brain happily uses some. That's right, thinking burns carbs. But there's a limit, so don't assume 'I'll just think myself skinny'!

When the brain has drunk enough glucose, what happens to the rest? It carries on floating, seeing if anyone else needs any. It's like someone selling hotdogs and soda in a football stadium. It keeps floating. And floating.

But carbs can't float around forever. Walking down steep stadium steps is dangerous, and so is having too much glucose in your blood. Your body must make a decision. It's *this* decision that helps make some people skinny, and keeps others, fat.

The floating carbs must find a new home, fast. There are two homes to choose from. Muscle cells, where carbs get stored and

145

easily used later. Or fat cells, where carbs get turned into fat, and sometimes never get used!

Don't underestimate this. It's possibly the main reason that some people seem to be able to 'eat anything' and *still* not get fat. They naturally get rid of any leftover carbs by storing them temporarily in muscle. You can be the same by mimicking exactly what their body does.

How? We become the shepherd of excess carbs! And it's really simple, we just need to *move*. **Movement makes the surfaces of muscles more absorbent to carbs.** If you like, movement turns muscles into a *very* dry sponge.

When the body has been made to move, the hormone insulin works brilliantly, and helps muscles suck up excess carbs like a *Dyson* in a dusty desert.

This is what you want. But what happens if you don't do *any* movement and overeat carbs? Annoyingly, the surfaces of fat cells are always like a dry sponge, and always ready to get fatter. Why? Because our genes *always* worry about running out of food!

The only way to defeat our body's paranoia, is to move. This sends your body a message, 'hey, I'm a physical girl and I'm going to use these carbs soon, so don't you *dare* make me fatter'! **Movement makes muscle cells *better* than fat cells at absorbing carbs.**

This whole process is **hunting**. Movement is your body out there in the wild, searching around for food. Our genes might be 2,000,000 years old, but they haven't forgotten where they came from! **You hunt, and the body *revs* up.**

WAIT A MINUTE

So movement really turns the tables on those greedy fat cells, stopping them from gobbling up carbs and turning them into fellow fatties. But it gets better. All you have to do is **wait** a minute. Well, wait a few minutes actually.

After moving around, your body is sitting there, ready to deal with that extra slice of bread you just *couldn't* resist! But the bread isn't showing up. The body is confused. It's thinking, 'we've been hunting, surely we caught something?'.

The longer you wait, the more the body panics. Maybe it thinks your fellow hunters have stolen whatever you caught (e.g. lion, dinosaur, pasta). And in this panic, there is magic! It decides right there and then, to help your muscles.

The longer you wait after moving, the longer your body keeps burning fat, and the longer your body panics. It reasons that any spare carbs unwanted by your brain, must get stored in muscle to power another hunt.

It does this by boosting all kinds of **enzymes**. They're chemicals that speed up a process. In this case, it boosts an enzyme which helps you pull any excess carbs into muscle. It's called **glycogen synthase**. Names is for tombstones baby, so forget it!

All you need to know, is that waiting after you 'hunt', gets the body working on your side. At the same time, our old pal insulin is also hanging around, desperate to get food out of the blood, and into the cells who want it baddest.

Some of you might be thinking that it's good to wait for hours and hours. Nope. If you give your body no food for a *very* long time, it might start to eat you. Don't panic, you don't just stand and dissolve like the witch in *The Wizard of Oz!*

But gradually, starvation leads to muscle breakdown. Bits of them are sliced off and sent to your liver, who reluctantly turns them into energy. **Losing muscle like this will make you weak and slow you down**. This is how your body prevents you getting into more mischief.

So, we need to **hunt** (move), and we need to **wait** (wait!), *for a bit*. The question is how much of each? 15 minutes is the minimum amount of time to 'hunt' (move). This forces your body to take notice.

And roughly 15 minutes is the minimum amount of time you need to 'keep the meter running' (wait). This makes your body boost enzymes that will encourage muscles to suck up carbs after a meal (and stop those arrogant fat cells from feeling swell!).

HOW TO USE YOUR POM POMS

Everyone can benefit from the chemical changes that happen from this hunt and wait trick. I've written down the minimums for each group. Everyone shares the last pre-meal **pom 3**, a 15 minute hunt *followed* by a 15 minute wait.

The best way to make these sessions work, is to choose some movement that's easy to stick to. For most people, that doesn't mean going to a gym. You could use some home gym stuff if you want, but even a quick and simple walk is perfect.

WAVE

pom 2 (before meal 2) 15 minute hunt, 15 minute wait

pom 3 (before meal 3) 15 minute hunt, 15 minute wait

BLAZE

pom 2 (before meal 2) 15 minute hunt, 30 minute wait

pom 3 (before meal 3) 15 minute hunt, 15 minute wait

QUAKE

pom 2 (before meal 2) 30 minute hunt, 30 minute wait

pom 3 (before meal 3) 15 minute hunt, 15 minute wait

It's important to realize that **the hunting and the waiting are equally important**. Each forces your body to change the way it has responded to food in the past. Within a week of doing this, your body's entire *chemistry set* will be boosted.

Now, I'm not giving you a licence to raid the refrigerator, but these small shifts of timing help your body work as it was originally meant to. **Hunting and waiting are part of *your* ancient DNA**, and tapping into this will cause some seriously desirable physical changes.

The total amount of calories used in these sessions *isn't* the most important thing, although burning calories always helps. It's actually the unique timing that turns your body's chemical and biological clock back 2,000,000 birthdays.

So if you were to do your pom 1, pom 2 and pom 3 as one giant workout, the effect wouldn't be as good as splitting them in three. You'd burn similar calories in total, but the changes to your biochemistry would be nothing like as powerful.

And **for many who choose their worst foods at night, pom 3 is a life saver**. It gives your body a fighting chance of extracting nutrients, and sending any unused stuff into the right homes (carbs into muscle cells instead of fat cells).

RUN FORREST, *RUN*

Any form of hunting (movement) will help you get skinny. In the section on movement itself, I talked about how to plan your sessions. For most of you, your morning pom 1 just needs to be about doing the target time, and waiting after.

That first session is also best done with a form of movement that involves as much muscle as possible, so that after sleep, you'll burn maximum calories. But for the other two quick sessions, it's cool to be a bit more relaxed. How?

By finding forms of movement that you really enjoy, to the point that you don't even realize that you're doing them. Making them different from your morning means that you're less likely to get bored. Remember, **movement *is* what it *is***.

As you get skinnier, you might find some new energy that you never thought possible. If you get this excitement, and you want to use it, don't hold back! For some people, that could mean doing a more intense form of movement.

Often by afternoon or evening, the body is much warmer than earlier. Our lungs are more able to fill with air later in the day too. Your pom 1 might feel like it has warmed your entire system up. You'll sense a *looseness*.

So, if you're out and about, and have an extra chunk of strange energy, use that chunk! Your body is simply adapting to your new demands. Whenever you have the energy, run *Forrest*, run! **Never 'save' energy up**.

GET THE SKINNY ON...

OMG 6 Your body is designed to hunt and wait before it eats

OMG 5 Movement sessions make muscles soak up excess carbs better

OMG 4 Waiting after movement sessions boosts extra chemicals to help this

OMG 3 Movement sessions don't just work because you burn calories in them

OMG 2 Even just 15 minutes hunting and waiting will ignite your ancient DNA

OMG 1 All hunt and wait sessions are equally important

OMG ! Make sure whenever you eat you hunt and wait first!

BECOME A HEAVY METAL CHICK

What do you know about lifting weights? Perhaps that guys do it, you enjoy watching them do it, and that if you do it, you'll turn into one? Wrong, wrong and wrong! If you really want to get *the OMG reaction*, **you need to do weights**.

Why? I'm going to give you at least 5 top reasons. If you've already made your mind up that you *don't* need to do weights, unmake it! You'll be able to get a great body without them. But it won't ever be *fantastic*. Which does Madam prefer?

GET BIGGER, GET SMALLER

Doing weights will help you shrink your overall size. Sounds unlikely, but it's true. Some of you might be reading that and thinking, 'I've tried weights, and they just made me bigger'. Maybe they did, but that's only in the beginning. How?

When people first use weights, they build a *tiny* bit of muscle, *quickly*. Not enough to make them look like an Olympic gymnast, but enough to notice a difference. At the same time, they don't lose body fat so fast (the wrong diet). They get bigger!

This is a temporary illusion. Imagine looking down at your body from directly above. See the center core of your legs. Bones. Around them are muscles, and then fat and then skin. If you make the muscles a bit bigger, they push the rest outwards, making you think that everything's grown *way* more than it really has.

Quitting weights is a mistake. Muscle is the stuff that helps you *get* skinny and *stay* like that, all without starving yourself. Even if you're a girl who gains muscle bulk quickly, you must realize that just as quickly, the bulking will slow down. Dramatically.

So, what's the big deal with muscle anyway? Let me tell you about your body's fat stores first. They're lazy. They just sit there and hang out on the porch! Body fat stores don't burn calories. **Body fat *is* calories**.

But your muscles are different. They're like a bunch of restless kids, always needing attention. And by that, I mean they *need* calories. Here's an obvious statement: you can't move without moving a muscle, and muscles run on calories.

Another obvious statement: if you have more muscle, you'll burn more calories. Science estimates that each pound of muscle burns about 50 calories per day. Yet all this 'new' science stuff is old news, and misses the point (especially for girls).

Why? Because it's that thing we don't do. Theory! More muscle *would* burn more calories. But that's looking at it from completely the wrong angle. Scientists, if you're secretly reading this book, be truly wise owls and rotate you heads around my way!

As a girl, building lots of muscle *isn't* likely. Magazines, books and science journals are full of well-meaning but dumb advice about girls building muscle. Most girls just don't. But **most girls do *lose* lots of muscle on diets**. Scientists, you can rotate your heads back now.

THE HORRORS OF 28 DAYS LATER

In fact in almost all changes of diet, we lose muscle. Every pound of muscle you lose is 50 fewer calories to play with. '50 calories?' you scoff! How about losing 5 pounds of muscle? People lose that amount all the time.

This lowers metabolism by 5 lots of 50 calories, or 250 calories per day. 28 days later, you would have burned 7000 *less* calories. Enough to gain 2 lbs. This is the scary truth behind what makes dieters *plateau* (a fancy way of saying weighing scales stop being nice!).

We only reach a plateau if we're doing something wrong. For most people, **a diet only stops working if basic principles are broken or ignored**. Losing muscle is something that many dieters ignore, or actually don't even realize.

Every ounce of muscle you lose reduces your ability to burn calories. And it also scares the body. We need muscle to get around in this world, literally! If the body senses a loss of muscle, it slows everything down to save itself.

Most changes of diet make you lose muscle. This is bad. Muscle is your friend, because it helps you deal with food properly. Don't lose your friend, do weights!

So, while it's unlikely that you'll ever become a pro wrestler, you need to train like one! **Your goal is to maintain muscle while you're dieting**, and therefore keep your metabolism stoked up to the max. It takes very little effort, and it's worth it.

BE FIRM

Once You Start Losing Body fat, you will start to *look* firmer. And that happens because you're losing fat, and allowing the skin to shrink closer towards your muscles. But the truth is, your muscles themselves haven't changed that much.

By increasing your daily movement, some of your muscles will get a bit firmer. But not much, and nowhere near the same firmness you get from doing weights. **Weights make all muscles firm**, to look at *and* to squidge!

BECOME UNBREAKABLE

When the first astronauts came back from space, they never expected to feel how they did. After stepping out of their space craft, they collapsed. This wasn't just joy! These super fit guys had suddenly become extremely weak just by vacationing in space. Why?

Space, unlike *Earth*, has no gravity. Just think of gravity as pressure pushing down on you. Literally like someone pressing down on your shoulders. Or if you like, it's the thing that stops you from leaping over tall buildings!

Hanging around our *Moon* caused the astronaut's muscles and bones to adapt to their new surroundings. They got *weaker*.

The easiest way to copy what happens in space, is to lie in bed, doing nothing. This is exactly how *NASA* tests their space pilots against this!

As you diet and reduce your body weight, your muscles and your bones will have less reason to stay strong. This is why lighter women often have more bone and muscle weakness than heavier women. And pretty soon, you *will* be lighter!

Weight training artificially puts bones under pressure and makes them stronger as a result. Don't worry, they don't grow outwards! They get tougher inside. Keeping your bones strong will help you throughout life, and keep you injury-free.

SHAPE YOUR DESTINY

At the moment you're born, and I mean 9 months *before* you roll onto the planet, your basic shape is decided. That means that your genes have a plan. This plan contains your bone lengths, and the positioning of all your fat and muscle cells.

But that's just the beginning. **With weight training, you can really change your shape**. You can't completely change your proportions, but you definitely can make everything look more even. And that makes anyone look better.

CARB SHEPHERD

When you overeat carbs, you create problems. Too many carbs floating around in the blood is dangerous. Because of this, your body releases insulin to take the excess and put it somewhere safe. I know you know already! There are 2 safe places.

Muscle cells or *fat* cells. If your muscles work as they're supposed to, they'll suck up most of the carbs, and use them soon. But if your muscles don't work well, all the carbs float into fat cells, where they'll be made *into* more body fat.

Obviously, we want excess carbs to hook up with muscle cells. Any form of movement helps this process, but pumping iron is king. **Weight training makes all your muscles boost their ability to absorb all excess carbs.**

By now you've got enough reasons to give weight training a proper go. All of them will boost your chances of getting a killer body. **Even if you don't care about the health benefits, weight training keep fat loss going.** Sold? Great! Here's the hows.

HOW OFTEN TO HIT THE WEIGHTS

Good news first, especially if you're still dreading the thought of doing weights. **You just need to train muscles with weights at least once every 10 days.** That's it! It may sound bizarre, but it's enough to do the trick.

Magazines and books often tell girls to do complex weights routines 3 or more times *per week*. **This isn't necessary.** You mainly need to do weights to protect your muscles from shrinking. And that takes just 3 times *per month*.

And to do that, it's all about how *hard* you train, not how often. If you train hard, at least once every 10 days, you tell the body, 'I need my muscles to stick around'. And that's what your body does for you. So, *how hard* is hard?

HOW HARD TO HIT THE WEIGHTS

This is important. So many articles are written with neat little pictures of girls holding baked bean cans for dumbbells. This will only ever tell your body to get good at lifting baked bean cans, and that's hardly different from everyday life!

By now, you'll have realized that **weights won't make you muscle bound**. So, you really can go for it and train hard. And if you're lifting weights, hard is something that's hard to do more than 10 times.

Again, the media tends to be a bit bamboozled when it comes to recommending the ideal number of repetitions (*reps* for short). They usually talk about doing 15 or 20 or even higher. And that's utter nonsense!

If you can lift something 20 times, it *must* be pretty light. And that's useless at stimulating your muscles, especially if you don't train them every day. But what about those who say doing lots of reps burns lots of fat?

Nonsense ditto! To burn *lots* of fat, movement must use *lots* of muscle, e.g. walking. Doing that uses at least 10 major muscles *every* rep (i.e. every step), and therefore it's like doing over 1000 reps a minute. **Doing 20 reps for fat loss is like walking 2 steps!**

Training with light weights for high reps doesn't stimulate your muscles, and it's not enough to directly burn fat. Count high numbers for games of hide and seek! **For weights, keep your reps to 10 or less. When 10 is easy, make it harder.**

WHERE TO HIT THE WEIGHTS

A gym is best, but don't panic if that's totally out of the question (there are four alternatives). A gym is great because there's lots of variety to prevent you getting bored, and it's often the place where you will train with gusto.

It's also safe, once you know what you're doing. It can be quite motivating to see others working out, especially if you're used to being around people who don't naturally inspire you. And if buff people scare you, find somewhere quiet.

You don't need to join a gym, as most places will let you pay for a guest workout. Remember, training hard just once every 10 days, that's 3 times per month, is enough to keep your muscles ticking over and fat loss nicely revved up.

So, what about those who just *can't* face using a commercial gym, or who can't afford it, or are perhaps too young? Well, there are other choices. Here's a few of the best for you to consider:

CIRCUIT TRAINING CLASSES

Most gym classes are way too soft! They're great for when you just want to chill or even want to hang out with people. But to help protect *your muscles* from being way too soft, one type of class stands out above all the others. **Circuit Training**.

This is where small pieces of equipment are placed around a fitness studio, and an instructor shouts at you to use them! Often classes are to music, which helps get you moving. The movements tend to be varied, and this is great for muscles.

Circuit training is half like weight training in a hurry, and half like going for a run. This combination is great at boosting your calorie burning too. A good class will be very tough, so start with something easier but move up when you feel ready.

There are now outdoor versions of circuit training held in parks and open spaces all over the world. These so-called 'park fitness' or 'army training' classes are great, but only if they're hard for your muscles (and not just for your lungs).

PILATES CLASSES

Joseph Pilates was a self-taught fitness guru who designed a training system to strengthen and control the body (modestly called **Pilates**!). It's had a boom recently, and for dieters, it's very useful as it concentrates on really using muscle.

There are many styles, with some using machines and others using just a floor mat, but they all help you prevent muscle loss. The advantage of Pilates is that most places will let anyone do it, even if you're 12.

YOGA

Some see **yoga** as a gentle fadult pursuit, or maybe just a 5,000 year old stretching routine! Sometimes this is true, but yoga *can* be tough on muscles, and available to almost anyone. That makes it great for our use.

There are many styles of yoga, but it's not important for you to get caught up in all that. You just need to find the toughest form of yoga you can. And by tough, I mean one which makes your muscles feel like they've been to war and back!

As with Pilates, and even circuit training, yoga doesn't have to be about doing high speed movement. **We are choosing things that tell our muscles to stick around**. By doing that, you keep your metabolism high, and you always progress.

A NOTE ABOUT CLASSES

There is one very cool benefit of doing classes. They *make sure* that you work your muscles hard. All you have to do is turn up, and someone will 'help' you! Sometimes we all need a kick. If a class feels easy, find a tougher class.

Classes make it simple to keep track of how often you're working your muscles. Although once every 10 days is the minimum, there's nothing wrong with you doing something hard once every 7 days, i.e. doing a hard, fun, regular class, once a week.

Finally, classes are social. Training by yourself at home, or in a gym where you feel alone or intimidated might make you give up. If you find a class where you fit in (it may take a few weeks to become 'trusted' by regulars), you'll probably keep going back to it.

TRAINING IN YOUR BEDROOM

If you've got very little money, or you really can't face venturing out into public yet, it's better that you **do something instead**

of nothing. You can't get much more personal than training in your own bedroom.

At the very minimum, you'll need to get yourself **a set of adjustable dumbbells**. In the beginning, you might even need someone to carry these into your bedroom! They're simply a pair of small metal bars, on which you add circular weight discs.

And you need them to be *adjustable*, because your strength naturally improves the more you use them. If you buy weights which are fixed in terms of how heavy they are, you'll out-grow them. Another reason why baked bean cans are useless!

Training in your bedroom has advantages. It's quiet, you can focus, and you can do it when it suits you. The main problems are the opposite of these, i.e. it's easy to get distracted, and you might just never get into the habit.

Training alone can be dangerous too, so that's something you've got to be aware of. Dumbbells are generally impossible to get trapped underneath, but they still can cause injury if you drop them (and if you do that, your fat-loss secret will be out with a loud thud!).

The main thing is that you do some kind of all over, tough training for your muscles at least once every 10 days.

I'm going to put an example of a routine at the end of the section. It's impossible to explain exercises with pictures or even videos. You need to *do* them. For some, you might want to use a trainer once or twice to show you things.

HOW TO PICK A TRAINER

If you're not sure, *ask*. We hear that phrase all time. And despite hearing it, we rarely ever ask. Starting at school, our arms seem to be glued to our sides, and by the time we get confident enough to speak up, the bell's rung! Don't let the bell ring on your success.

If you want to use a trainer to help you learn some weight training techniques, you need to get a good one. And I'm not giving you these tips to save you money. You need to learn the techniques fast, then get on and use them!

Having a trainer might make you look cool, but what's cooler is if you reach your goals. Pick their brains, listen up well, and then work super hard. Find what motivates you instead of relying on a trainer to be your drill instructor.

PICK A TRAINER WHO...

- Can teach you the right techniques in 2 hours or less

- Focuses on you and doesn't start speaking to others

- Listens to your goals instead of giving you random or samey advice

- Never leans on pieces of equipment

- Doesn't use their phone in the gym

- Doesn't have a pushy personality

- Has brains and not just *Taylor Lautner's* bod!

If you can get someone who can do *all* of that, it's worth booking one session with them. Remember, you just want to learn how to do the movements well, and then work them hard, once every ten days. **Three times per month**. *Simple.*

If you're already confident with using a gym, or if you're determined to teach yourself, I've put some basic bits of advice below. We're all a little bit different, but these movements are a great place to start.

SIMPLE SAMPLE WEIGHTS ROUTINE

DUMBBELL SQUATS (2 SETS OF BETWEEN 5 AND 10 REPS)

These work your thigh muscles. That's the front of them, the back of them, and your butt! They're often described as a basic movement. That's not true, because it's the hardest one to get right. Learn to do this movement perfectly.

It will stimulate half of your body to get better at absorbing excess carbs, burn more fat all the time, and it will give you a much better overall shape. As I said, all the movements deserve more than pictures so I won't attempt to do that here.

DUMBBELL SHOULDER PRESS (2 SETS OF BETWEEN 5 AND 10 REPS)

This looks like an old-fashioned caveman movement! It involves having a dumbbell in each hand, and pushing them up overhead. This movement works so much muscle, and that will really benefit your overall shape and fat loss.

A brilliant version is to start with your hands at your sides, curl up both dumbbells, and then push them up over your head. This makes sure that the fronts of your arms get a nice workout before the backs of your arms help push the weight up.

It's a movement that also works your shoulders, your chest and even your spinal muscles, which have to work hard just to keep you balanced. Always do this movement standing, as that's actually safer and better for making muscles work.

DUMBBELL ROWS (2 SETS OF BETWEEN 5 AND 10 REPS)

Your back muscles, even if you're small, cover a big portion of your upper body. You need to protect this from shrinking when dieting, as all that muscle helps you deal with the food you eat every day. Dumbbell rows are great.

Again, it sounds like a simple movement, but you have to do it properly to get the best from it. You bend over at the waist, almost like doing a bow, and pick up a dumbbell in each hand. And then, you imagine that you're starting a chainsaw!

I mean, you pull your arms back like you were rowing a boat. This must be done carefully, so you don't damage your lower back. It tones all the muscles you can't see, and also the backs of your arms (which others *can* see easily!).

SWISS BALL CRUNCHES (2 SETS OF BETWEEN 5 AND 10 REPS)

This is also known as a **stability ball**, and if you've ever used one, you'll know why! They're hard to do anything on, and that's the point. They make all muscles, especially those in your midsection, work super hard.

Again, like squats, they're seen as basic, but that's not really true. Swiss balls look like big plastic bouncy toys. You need to get the right size, and that probably means somewhere between 21 and 25 inches (55 to 65 centimeters).

If you do crunches on these things, they are *miles* better than doing crunches on the floor. Floor crunches can be done for endless reps, because they're too easy. And as you might realize by now, doing hundreds to burn body fat won't work either.

Swiss ball crunches start with your abs stretched, which makes it difficult. Muscles are like rubber bands. The more you stretch them, the harder they ping back. Doing crunches like this will tone your tummy amazingly, and boost your confidence.

A FEW POINTERS ON DOING WEIGHTS MOVEMENTS

Obviously, I've made little attempt to describe these movements in detail. If I did, it might convince you that's all you need to know. That would be just like seeing a crap trainer! You need to see them done properly, and then learn them yourself.

All weights movements need to be done at a medium speed. Too fast risks injury and also makes muscles work less. Doing movements too slow means you'll probably need to use light weights, and taking too long could make you lose concentration.

Your first lot of reps (called a **set**) can be a little lighter if you want, to warm up the muscles. But still, **never get into the**

habit of doing more than 10 reps. Doing super light weights *doesn't* help muscles, and it *doesn't* burn fat.

If you can't get 5 reps, it's a bit heavy. If you can cruise past 10, it's a bit light. Stay between 5 and 10 reps. Become brilliant at counting numbers 5, 6, 7, 8, 9, 10!

After you've done your first set of up to 10 reps, you need to rest for a bit. **Rest for 3 minutes**. It might seem like ages, but if you're pushing hard enough, the rest is needed for your muscles to work hard during the next set. It's not a race! Rest.

You generally don't need to do any special warm up for doing weights, unless you're very cold. If you are cold, even moving around randomly for a few minutes will help. Warm muscles work much better than freezing cold ones.

Your muscles are rubber bands. If they're cold, they're less springy. And you want them springy! Springy muscles are strong. To get that, move! Blood is warm, and when it washes around, it heats muscles like a hairdryer over a rubber band.

Because you only need to do your weights once every 10 days, it doesn't really matter when you do them. Ideally though, it would be good to work out *just before* your second or third meal (you can treat it as a *hunt and wait* session, and leave a 15 minute gap after). Doing this will help your muscles repair.

When you train with weights, your muscles develop tiny tears. I mean so tiny you'd need a microscope to see them! But these tears need fixing. Protein helps that, and eating some close to a workout gives them a nice recovery boost.

167

The take-home message of this huge section seems complicated, but it's not. **If you do weights at least once every 10 days, you'll get a fantastic body, skinny and with shape**. Work your muscles hard and they'll love you back.

GET THE SKINNY ON...

OMG 6 To get toned all over you need to do weights all over

OMG 5 Weights save muscle and muscle burns your calories

OMG 4 Weights build shape, bones and help you deal with excess carbs

OMG 3 Do weights intensely enough to challenge your muscles

OMG 2 Gym's are great but so are tough classes (circuit training, yoga and Pilates)

OMG 1 Even training in your bedroom with dumbbells will help lots

OMG ! Find a way to train your muscles hard 3 times per month!

PARTY TRICKS WITH BALLOONS

You might have read the last section, and wondered if there was anything more you could do for your stomach. There's something funny about how we treat our middles. We treat them to everything! I mean, we often work harder on them than any other bit.

Most people think that to get an amazing tummy, you need to be really skinny, be 'born like that', or spend time doing thousands of sit-ups every day. How much of this is true? To get an OMG reaction to your middle, here's the rub.

A NICE PAIR OF GENES

Your genetics are decided by your parents, including how your stomach looks. It gets decided 9 months *before* you step out into the world. You're thinking, 'I can't believe no one asked me what I wanted for my zero birthday'! Naughty parents.

At that moment, nature throws the dice. Depending on pure chance, you'll either have lots of fat cells in your middle, or not so many. You can't change this. But it's not really a big deal, because **all fat cells can be shrunk** down.

And if you have lots of fat cells in one area, you usually have *less* in another. The rarest type of genes are those people who have their fat cells spread evenly over the body. But even they still need to eat and move well (or they'll simply be *evenly* fat!).

SIT UP AND NOTICE NOTHING

If you've ever done thousands of sit-ups or crunches, you may have noticed a few things. Your stomach may have got firmer. That's because you've been working the main muscle at the front of your tummy (it's called the **rectus abdominis**, a.k.a **six-pack**).

You may have also noticed that you *didn't* lose much fat in the area. That's because sit-ups or similar movements involve a *tiny* amount of muscle, and therefore only use up a *tiny* amount of energy (body fat).

The lines on your stomach which make up a six-pack, are tendons. They actually protect you in case one 'chunk' gets injured. Seeing them will mainly depend on your level of body fat. To get that low, just keep using what you've learnt so far.

Some notice that working out or being skinny doesn't make their stomach truly flat. And that's because most movements don't work a special muscle that our eyes can't see. And if we can't even *see* it, being skinny doesn't much help it.

It's called the **transversus**. By working it, you won't really get more six-pack lines, but it will become excitingly flat. Yes, excitingly. It will flatten and flatter you like wearing a Victorian corset, *without* the pain! How can we train this hidden gem?

AND . . . BREATHE OUT

By blowing up balloons! It sounds weird, but it works, and works quickly. If a super flat tummy sounds appealing to you, spend some time doing this. It's worth the effort. So, what do you need?

Balloons! If you can, buy a few different types, and don't worry about what's written on them! Try to get some which are easy to blow up (to get used to), and some which are a little more difficult. Don't expect the sales assistant to know which are which! Just buy some.

To use balloon exercises, **wait a few hours after eating**. When we eat, our stomach, which can't hold much food, fills up quickly. If you feel bloated, breathing hard is difficult. And you will need to breathe hard!

If you have high blood pressure, a hernia, stomach ulcer, or lower back problems, it could be dangerous to use balloons. If you're not sure, ask a doctor before you try them. These are muscles that you probably haven't worked hard for a while. Possibly never!

It's important to do the exercises without too many clothes on. A tight belt or pair of jeans, or any clothes that make you feel *squeezed* are bad for breathing. Whip 'em off and on to the floor! And if possible, always stand in front of a mirror.

And it is important *to stand*, and not sit. Humans were designed to stand, move or lay flat. The in-between bit (sitting) makes breathing more difficult. So, get your balloons, get comfortable, and stand tall.

Starting with the easiest balloon you can (usually the softest and most flexible), bring the balloon to your mouth, and blow! It helps if you keep your elbows quite high, about the same level as your face.

When a balloon is new, it's difficult to blow up. I'm sure you know this, especially if you've ever been asked to inflate some for a party and failed miserably! So, on the first breath, push hard, but go steady.

Once you've puffed fully, take it away from your face, and let the air out. Take another deep breath, and go again. If you're in front of a mirror, when you're breathing *in*, check to see that the bottom corners of your ribcage are expanding as wide as possible.

It's good to do these exercises once per day, and rest the next day. For example, do them on Monday, Wednesday, Friday, Sunday, Tuesday and so on. You don't need to do them every day, and besides, you'll need to buy a suspicious amount of balloons!

Blowing up a balloon, is like lifting a weight with your arms, i.e. **you're working a muscle**. When muscles work against a force like a weight, or a balloon's *stretch*, they need rest to recover and get stronger.

But in the first week, you can do them a bit more. This lets your body wake-up the transversus and helps get it ready to be used more often. Try to stick to this first week routine (but don't panic if you forget or miss a day).

When you blow air out with force, you will naturally take a bigger than normal breath in. This **deep breathing may make you**

dizzy or sick. If this happens, stop. We're not trying to personally prevent a hot air balloon from crashing! *Rest* for a few minutes.

The best time for balloons is before bed. At night, our lung capacity (our ability to breathe) is at a peak. Plus, deep breathing can boost growth hormone, the chemical that makes us skinnier, firmer, and have better skin.

PARTY TRICK WARM-UP PLAN

Day 1 – Aim to blow the balloon up 10 times

Day 2 – Aim to blow the balloon up 12 times

Day 3 – Aim to blow the balloon up 14 times

Day 4 – Aim to blow the balloon up 16 times

Day 5 – Aim to blow the balloon up 18 times

Day 6 – Do nothing, you need to rest!

Day 7 – Do nothing again, you still need to rest!

Once you've completed this warm-up week, your muscles will be awake! It's quite possible that even after a week, your stomach will be *much* flatter. From then on, you can stick to a maintenance plan for the rest of *Six Weeks To OMG*.

PARTY TRICK MAINTENANCE PLAN

- Blow up balloons every alternate night

- Blow up the balloon **20** times

- Rest for **3** minutes

- Blow up the balloon another **20** times

- Chuck the balloon away (i.e. use a new one each time)

BLOW OUT DAY

After 6 weeks, it's still great to blow balloons once per week, for as long as the world makes balloons! It will keep your entire middle flat and strong. That will then protect you from all kinds of injuries for life (including back aches).

At first, you might find blowing up balloons weird, boring, and easy to forget. Give it a chance. For a few days, your tummy might be sore. After a week, it won't. After two, it will look different. And after 6, you'll count OMGs instead of breaths!

GET THE SKINNY ON...

OMG 6 To see your stomach definition you must be skinny overall

OMG 5 To get a flat stomach you must work your transversus muscle

OMG 4 Blowing up balloons works this muscle better than anything

OMG 3 Deep breathing also boosts growth hormone which burns fat

OMG 2 Blow up balloons every alternate night for 6 weeks

OMG 1 When you finish your plan do them once per week

OMG ! Go out and buy some balloons right now!

STUCK IN THE MIDDLE

Oh yes, another section on the tummy! In the last few years, scientists have stated that fat around your middle was 'more dangerous than fat anywhere else'. Guess what's more dangerous?

That statement! We'll talk **belly fat** in a tick, but giving it super kudos makes people, especially women, believe that they're healthy if they don't have any. Wrong. **All excess fat is dangerous**. Yep, even *that* bit you're subconsciously squeezing now!

So, what's the deal about belly fat? Using high-tech scans, scientists discovered that fat above the belt is physically wrapped around nearby organs. The guys and girls in white coats hide this already hidden fat behind a strange name, **visceral fat**.

Visceral fat acts differently compared to fat under our skin (called **subcutaneous fat**). Under the skin fat just makes us soft, pushes up blood pressure, heart disease and maybe cancer. Pretty safe then!

But belly fat causes stuff like diabetes, inflammation (e.g. arthritis), and heart disease too. Why? Because **visceral fat cells leak out irritating chemicals**. This irritation starts slowly, and gets worse.

In the beginning, it worsens asthma (if you have it), gives you blotchy skin, and even increases how acid-like your body feels.

But it can get really bad. Irritation from fat cells makes the body attack *itself*.

Left unchecked, it creates painful joints. Do you ever wake up in the morning and feel sore or achy without reason? That could be your fat cells leaking out these irritating chemicals overnight.

What's exceedingly dangerous is irritation that affects your heart and arteries. If you annoy them, you could develop blockages in your pipes. It's a slow process, but in a way, that's what makes it deadly.

You can reduce irritation by eating natural food, and by boosting your intake of omega-3 fats (found in supplements and fish). But they can only do so much. Want a better way? Get skinny and clear out those leaky fat cells for good!

Having a big belly also makes insulin go wrong. And remember, we depend on insulin to clear up after having a carb party. **If you're a girl with a waist more than 35 inches, or a guy who's beyond 40 inches, your insulin might be 'broken'**. Fix it by getting skinny.

Most of us talk about where we store fat in strangely polite ways, using phrases like 'apple' and 'pear'. I love the way we use fruit to describe human shape! As I said earlier though, this kind of attitude misses the point.

And the point is, **all excess body fat is proof that we're doing something wrong**. This can't be denied. So, what's the solution? Firstly, keep following this book in general and get skinny fast. And secondly, read the next chapter.

GET THE SKINNY ON...

OMG 6 Belly fat is fat wrapped around your organs

OMG 5 It leaks irritating chemicals into your blood

OMG 4 They cause joint pain, rashes, asthma, heart problems and diabetes

OMG 3 Belly fat also makes your muscles worse at dealing with carbs

OMG 2 Until you lose belly fat, dietary omega-3 fat can reduce irritation

OMG 1 If your waist is over 35" (over 40" for guys) get skinny fast

OMG ! Just focus on fat loss in general and belly fat will go!

FAT AND MISERABLE

If you look up 'visceral' in a dictionary, it probably won't mention a type of belly fat. It might say something like 'affecting inward feelings'. In fancy talk, if we say something's visceral, it means that we feel it *inside*.

Science has found that our *inner feelings* actually affect our *inner fat*. Stress raises a hormone called cortisol. And cortisol makes humans store more fat around the middle.

Isn't Mother Nature cruel? If she sees we're stressed about *being* fat, she releases a chemical that makes us even fatter. And then we get stressed again! How can we break this cycle? Stick around. But first, let me explain her actions.

JURASSIC SPARK

When you get stressed, whatever 'stress' means for you, you release **cortisol**. That's why geeks call it our 'stress hormone'. It dates back a few million years, and it exists to save us *from* stress. Confused?

If you were running from a dinosaur, you'd need some rapid energy. Body fat is a great fuel, but it needs lots of oxygen to burn. It's like a wooden log in a fire. You need to fan it with lots of air. You get lots of air during normal pace living.

When you're always on the run from dinosaurs, air's in pretty short supply. You move *way* more than you breathe. That's why breathing takes time to calm down after you've stopped moving (so-called, 'catching my breath'). Nervousness makes us breathe shallow too.

To move quick, you need quick energy. Carbs in the blood are like tissue paper and burn easily, perfect for a quick boost. The problem is, those prehistoric cave dwellers often lived miles away from their local carb palace, the *Kwik-E-Mart*.

But, they still had a mini *Kwik-E-Mart* inside them. Their *Liv-E-r Mart*. Okay I'll stop being smart, they still had their liver! *It* has stored carbs. Any spark of stress ignites your liver to empty its stored carbs into the blood, which helps you move miles from *the big beast*.

SPOT THE DIFFERENCE

What happens if your big beast isn't something you can escape from? What happens if your big beast, *your stress*, is mental? Well, the prehistoric wiring is still there, and **your brain can't tell the difference between mental and physical stress**.

This means that you could be sitting in class, in a traffic jam, or simply worrying about how fat you are, and you'd release the stress hormone cortisol. Slowly but surely, that empties out the liver's stored carbs into the blood.

And with no physical movement to power, that previously tucked away energy ends up *becoming* body fat. Logically, this conversion usually takes place close to the area where it started. I mean, **unused carbs released from the liver become fat in your nearby belly**.

Cortisol is a necessary hormone at times, but we were never designed to deal with purely mental stress. We are literally made to run away from stress.

Before I give you some ideas on how to deal with this stressful (!) new knowledge, I want to talk about something related. It's the thing that many of us do when we're *feeling* stressed. It's possibly the worst psycho-physical habit of the 20th and 21st century.

COMFORT EATING

The subtitle really says it all. Comfort. Through *eating*. We had 2,000,000 years of using food for fuel, and then in the tiniest blink of time, the last 100 years, we've turned it into something different. **Food has become a hug**.

We go for hugs when we're sad, hugs when we're nervous, and I believe this is the one that everyone's been underestimating, hugs when we're just *bored*. Hugs from food are more reliable than people, because unlike friends on *Facebook*, they're *never* offline!

Why are these food hugs *so* good? Dopamine. Remember it? It's our reward chemical. It makes us feel good, and it makes us want to get the feeling again. And again. And again. Did I mention again, again? Again!

And guess what food type produces the biggest dopamine rush? You got it. Way more than fat and way more than protein, carbs are *the rush*. And **man-made sugars are the crack cocaine of food**, i.e. the worst of the worst.

As you know by now, excess carbs in our diet also make us chunky. And feeling like a chunky monkey isn't good for self-esteem! In many of us, feeling like crap, makes us head back to the refrigerator, to eat more crap.

This pattern of *feeling crap* and *eating crap* is the worst addiction on the planet. Obesity is deadly, and yet feeding that addiction is available around the clock, and comes without fear of arrest. Well, maybe cardiac arrest.

Addiction problems are the same with all drugs. You need more and more to keep the same 'high'. In the case of food, problems don't just happen in the brain. Comfort eating slowly makes your muscles get worse at absorbing 'comfort'.

Your muscles will always struggle with carb addiction. If you keep blasting them with carbs, they will stop working properly. They literally become 'fed' up with carbs.

Insulin rockets in an attempt to hammer nutrients into faulty muscles that sit there with their arms crossed. Eventually, the organ that makes insulin, your pancreas, gives up. **Welcome to diabetes**. For the first time in human history, this can now *start* to happen in your teens.

You don't have to be one of them. Breaking addiction to food comes from a mixture of knowing that you're doing it, wanting to change, and getting so upset that you actually end up doing something about it. Step one, done.

Step two, get practical. Start eating those meals instead of snacks, even if it drives you mad for a few weeks. **Eating snacks is like seeing a drug dealer more often. You're much more likely to stay addicted. Get away from the snack ghetto**.

Movement helps stress, but not how experts think. Stress is rarely caused by not moving, so moving more isn't the magical cure they swear by. Here's a skinny but, *but* **moving definitely helps soak up excess carbs released** *from* **stress**.

HOW TO MAKE THE DINOSAURS EXTINCT AGAIN

The biggest step, and the only one, is to fix the root of your stress. **Food is not the cause of your stress, and cannot be its solution**. If you respect food as food, it won't come back to bite you in the butt!

Many of you will be stressed *because* you haven't got the perfect body yet. If this is you, you know the answer. Give it your all, right now. **Apply this book. Become an expert. Go get the body which you are truly destined for**.

Solving the cause of your stress is the only approach. Food gives us enjoyment as a bonus. There's a very old, but still very useful saying. We must eat to live, not live to eat. Same calories, different thinking.

If necessary, get help with whatever is making you feel stressed. If stress keeps you fat and fast-forwards you along the road towards mega obesity, you might eventually reach the stress-free place known as being dead.

When it comes to any kind of stress, don't just *block it out*. **Blocking it out is not dealing with it**. *It*, is still there, exactly like a program or app running in the background of your computer. These will whir away subconsciously and slow everything else down.

If this continues, every so often, *your* brain will freeze and you'll have to hit restart. And what form would the restart take? It always takes the path of some terrible, badly thought-out actions that just temporarily distract, and end up giving you way more pain.

Be smart. **Face your stress properly**. You may find that there's a solution well worth your attention. Your past 'tried to fix-it' attempts don't equal future ones. **Change is possible**. Know *what* you want fixed, *why* you want it fixed, and *go* fix it with your heart and soul.

Many experts praise meditation, hypnosis, NLP or even drugs. They're too complex to get into now. And whatever they say, they only work on the *result* of stress, not its true cause. Same as food really. If *Earth* had a comment on this subject, it might say something like:

Don't take it out on our food.

Thank you for your cooperation.

Alcohol. I'm not here to tell you whether to drink or not. That's between you and your liver! I *am* here to tell you, that it can increase the chance of having a belly. And no, it's not just guys who get beer belly.

Alcohol generally causes problems in women because they can't absorb it as well as men. This de-stressing tipple raises the stress hormone (!) cortisol, and may increase insulin too. Also, **alcohol contains plant versions of the hormone estrogen**.

It's not clear whether the extra estrogen makes females develop belly fat. In *theory* it wouldn't, but our hormone systems are so complex, it's tricky to predict how alcohol interacts with our body. If you drink, just be aware of this.

If you *have* to drink (assuming you're in the middle of the desert and the local oasis only sells alcohol), then it's smart to pick wisely. Alcohol *itself* contains 7 calories a gram. I'm not suggesting you count calories, but you must never consider it to be "just a chemical".

One problem with alcohol, is that it's rarely consumed by *itself*. Generally, to hide its chemical origins, it gets mixed with other stuff. Sugar, fat, and sometimes even protein is added to disguise a pure taste that could easily make your toes curl.

I'm going to assume that if you're interested in reading this section, it's because you drink alcohol to change your mental state, i.e. relax. If that's true, you might want to consider the drinks which get you to a relaxed state with the lowest amount of energy consumption.

HARD SPIRITS (LEAST LIKELY TO CAUSE ENERGY OVERCONSUMPTION)

Vodka, Whiskey, Brandy, Rum and Gin all tend to be similar in energy content, if you compare equal measure sizes. This is because they're close to being *pure alcohol*. In theory, drinking these undiluted ("neat" or "straight up") will mean total calorie content is kept low.

Put simply, hard spirits tend to get you "there" quickly (happy, on the floor, or perhaps both), reducing the likelihood of you over-indulging. Because of this, they're often *recommended* in diet books, or by weight-loss communities. But be careful. The modern trend is to mix these pure alcohols with sugar, often a carbonated soft drink. If this is your favorite tipple, just remember (*before* you go out!) to figure in the carb content you're glugging down. Liquid carbs still count, as do carbs consumed in near darkness!

Of course, the very latest trend is to mix hard spirits with artificially sweetened low or zero calorie drinks. Although this keeps energy content low while you're drinking, be aware that sweeteners, and alcohol itself, *could* increase cravings for *all* food at other times.

LIQUEURS (SOMEWHAT LIKELY TO CAUSE ENERGY OVERCONSUMPTION)

Liqueurs are alcoholic drinks that have been sweetened with either cream, herbs, fruits, spices, or even flowers. Their alcohol content is moderate to high, but they're sweet in taste, and this tends to quickly reduce energy overconsumption as the sweetness usually limits your chances of drinking too much.

WINES (QUITE LIKELY TO CAUSE ENERGY OVERCONSUMPTION)

Ancient grape juice, also known as wine, is a mixed bag. White wines tend to be higher in female hormones (estrogens) than red wines, and also contain less heart-healthy nutrients. Having said this, all wine, regardless of region or color, could become a problem.

The social nature of wine consumption (sharing a bottle), combined with moderate alcohol levels, lends itself perfectly to a gradual tidal wave of increased calories, before the brain knows what's got past the gate.

If wine is your thing, simply pick something you like, and forget choices based on it being "good for you". All alcohol has some *neurotoxicity* (it annoys the brain). Use smaller glasses, and try to not become your own bartender (i.e. sit near to the bottle!).

BEERS (VERY LIKELY TO CAUSE ENERGY OVERCONSUMPTION)

In this group, you can also include ales and ciders. The main ingredient is usually a cereal crop, like corn, barley or wheat, along with flavorings such as hops. Beers, like wine, have an alcohol content that varies wildly.

The trouble with beers is the way they get consumed: by the bottle, or in Europe especially, by the pint. Their high water content often masks the alcohol, allowing the drinker to heavily overindulge in excess energy.

On top of this, beer that contains hops, can be highly estrogenic. Plant estrogens, female sex hormones, can potentially mess with our own naturally produced hormones. This calorie and chemical excess must be respected, so be careful.

It's worth noting that *all* alcohol can affect your chances of getting skinny and healthy, simply due to how it makes you feel the next day. It's great to let your hair down, but be smart when it comes to something that could knock you off track completely.

LIGHTEN UP

Okay, let's get this one out of the bag. Smoking cigarettes causes a small (about 3 to 10%) increase in metabolic rate, which tends to last for 30 to 60 minutes. This probably comes from an increase in adrenaline hormones. They don't seem to affect appetite. Done.

And now for the *bad*. **Even if you increase your metabolic rate through smoking, you may end up using less energy overall, because you'll feel tired, and move less**. Our body needs lots of oxygen to function optimally, and smoking gets in the way of this.

Mechanically, the tar from cigarettes covers the insides of lungs, just as treacle would if you poured it over your fingers. This makes life difficult for the fingers *inside* your lungs, which are specifically designed to get air's oxygen into the body.

Chemically, the carbon monoxide in cigarettes stops oxygen being absorbed by the cells of the body. It's like they fill up all the seats on a bus, and good old oxygen has no where to sit. No oxygen, no fun, no zest for life. Carbon monoxide also makes breathing itself harder.

Psychologically, smoking does some weird things. **If you *feel* unhealthy because you're aware of your habit, you are much more likely to not care in general**. Anything that saps your motivation in life, is not good. With the right motive, you can move mountains.

Life is way too precious for you to be a slave to anything. Everyone has a beautiful mind. That's *everyone*. Minds only go ugly when one naughty idea takes control, and spins out of proportion. Why let cigarettes crack the whip and make demands you feel bad about?

Here's what I suggest. **Don't give up smoking**. This idea, common *everywhere*, is flawed thinking. You're not giving anything up. *Giving up* makes you think you're losing out on something. When someone takes something away, or we give it up, we just *crave* it back.

Get healthy and *free* yourself of smoking. That's the truth. **Set yourself *free***. Studies show that even death of a loved one through smoking doesn't tend to help the alive person. Even scary pictures or health films get ignored.

Use *whatever* helps *you*. The most powerful way to break free, is to have a cool bunch of people around you. **Support groups are the best way of putting tobacco to rest**. Motivation is the key, and fellow humans can be a brilliant way of perking you up.

Many of the problems we've discussed, fit into the nerdy description *Body Dysmorphic Disorder,* or BDD for short. In everyday language, it means worrying too much about your physical appearance, and that in itself is changing how you behave each day.

However it's described, it's not nice to be grabbed by it, and shaken around as if you're in the giant hands of a big, nasty monster. Scientists constantly argue (well, they "debate") about what it is, what causes it, and what to do about it.

BDD seems to take as many forms as there are different human personalities, but the common factor is *seeing* things differently, and then *feeling* bad about them. This problem with the outside sinks in to the inner thoughts, and that's what changes behaviors.

If you have a strong BDD, you might hate everything about your appearance. Some might just hate their skin, their hair, their nose, or perhaps in the context of this book, their body weight. Whether you hate one thing or a hundred things, it's still a problem to you.

Finding a fault logically leads to fixing the fault. You might frequently check yourself in the mirror, pull out your hair, scrub your skin, exercise non-stop, or do whatever *you* feel is necessary. At the extreme, you might fix the fault by avoiding society completely.

BDD often has its roots in childhood, or the time of opinions (when we become teens). Being teased is horrible, and even one throwaway comment can stick with us for years. Being abused is even worse. **The seeds of BDD, are always sown by others.**

I would like to take a moment to exclude the media from this. Although newspapers, websites, magazines, movies and TV shows put pressure on some people, they target *all* of us, and that's never the same as individuals saying or doing something nasty.

In parts of the world where the media doesn't exist, BDD still pops up. Criticism, from a nearby human, *directly* or *in passing*, is what sets it off. Jealousy, inaccuracy, or just not thinking before speaking will always be around in some form.

If you have BDD, there's no point in me telling you that you're a beautiful person with lots to say and give (even though I'm right), because you won't believe me. And I respect the fact that you don't believe me right now. I hope you will someday.

I will say this: love *can* heal everything, and whoever you are, in a world of 7,000,000,000 humans, there's a lid for every pot. Whether you're a lid or a pot, there's another one wandering around *looking* for *you*. Don't leave them wandering for too long.

If you're in really deep, and *need* help, it does exist. The absolute best bet is something called *CBT*, or *Cognitive Behavioral Therapy*. In non geek terms, that means doing stuff to change how your brain works (cognitive = brain, behavioral = change, therapy = doing stuff!).

If like me, you thought therapy sounded depressing, or dark, or something done by crazy people, *thought* again! We *all* need a check up from the neck up! Seriously, CBT is pretty cool. It's about seeing things differently, challenging old ideas, and thinking fresh.

In some ways, it's like life coaching. Many of us feel *shame* thinking about doing things for our brain. But why? I mean, look what you did for your body, you picked up this cheeky book! The brain deserves a workout too.

Seeing an expert is best, ideally by yourself. You *don't* have to tell anyone you're going. **Keep it a secret**. You might prefer to go to a group session, where you're not the focus of attention. And if you can't face the outdoors, order a book, or at least visit *Wikipedia* online!

As a species, us humans have done quite well. We can go on about our clever thumbs, amazing senses or brilliant brain, but what's made us *really* successful, is sharing stuff and finding solutions *together.* Go get some good old fashioned human help, today.

GET THE SKINNY ON...

OMG 6 Our ancient brain thinks mental stress is physical and releases cortisol

OMG 5 Cortisol tells your liver to empty stored carbs into the blood

OMG 4 If you don't use them up they get made into more body fat

OMG 3 Movement won't stop stress but helps absorbs stress-released carbs

OMG 2 Avoid man-made sugars (labeled '...ose') as they fuel comfort eating

OMG 1 Comfort eating from stress is a vicious cycle until you step off

OMG ! Find the true cause of your stress and start fixing it!

BEAUTY SLEEP

We've all been told that sleep is important. In fact, we're told that from a very early age. But sleep generally just gets talked about as something to do *when* you're tired, and to prevent you *being* tired. Old news. Want the fresh stuff?

In the past few years, we've got better at figuring out what sleep is really for. Some of these discoveries have only recently been made possible, and the info hasn't oozed out to those who need it most. Consider it oozed!

There are 5 solid reasons to get a fantastic sleep, and I mean fantastic. Don't dance over this chapter. That's what most books or experts do. Sleep is the thing we do for 30% of our lives, and we're way smarter than ignoring that. 30% not impressive? Think about it this way: **you could spend over 20 years lying in bed!** Yep, shocked me too!

SLEEP BOOSTS YOUR METABOLISM

Your metabolism is the rate at which your body uses energy (calories). Keeping it high makes your life easier (skinnier, healthier). The vast majority of people have a normal metabolism. And that includes *vast* people!

But when you change your diet, your metabolism often drops. This is your body trying to protect itself against change, as change is something the body does with caution. Give it time though, and it gets with the program.

In the meantime, you need to make sure that it's working as best as possible. To do that, you need to sleep. Properly. During sleep, your metabolism actually drops. It's like your computer going onto hibernate.

Your body takes a time-out. If you were planning to do something 2 billion times (like heart beats through life), you'd schedule slow-mo too! During this, things steadily reset. It's like pushing the *Jack* down in a *Jack-in-a-box*.

Sleep resets lots of chemicals. One of these, **thyroid hormone**, is very important for those who want to be skinny. Thyroid sets the speed of almost all chemical reactions in the body. What speed do we want? Full-speed ahead, *aye aye* captain, speed!

If you have a lovely *d-e-e-p* sleep, thyroid sinks low throughout the night, and then ROCKETS like *Jack* out-of-his-box first thing in the morning! This is exactly the pattern you want. When thyroid is high, your metabolism is on turbo boost.

But sleep badly, and your thyroid won't reset properly. Instead, it kind of stays permanently low. Enough to keep you going, but barely. You'll often feel colder after a bad night's sleep. *Skinny dipping*, first thing? Ouch!

This is because thyroid strongly affects your heat production. You could take your temperature daily if you wanted to prove this. A simpler way is to notice the extra goose bumps on your forearms around afternoon.

Although feeling cold seems *just* uncomfortable, it's a sign that your metabolism is seriously lowered. Remember that when you lose heat, you're getting rid of energy (calories). You need to sleep well to maximize this.

SLEEP MAKES YOUR SKIN, HAIR AND NAILS BEAUTIFUL

To get an OMG reaction, it helps to have great skin, hair and nails. Losing fat is a start, and so is eating smart. But what's even more important, is how good your 'factory' is at making cells. And sleep affects the factory!

During sleep, beauty cells are replaced. I mean, new skin, hair and nail cells get born in the deepest layers. It takes time (e.g. 2 to 3 weeks in skin) for cells to reach the top and be seen. Bad sleep isn't instantly obvious (apart from temporary dark circles).

Quite often you'll find people who have great skin, and hair, and nails. They're all made from the same stuff (protein plus sleep), so if you get that right, you tend to improve the three areas simultaneously.

If you keep sleeping badly, all the bad nights in the factory start to show up. Your skin might look uneven, heal badly and scar easily. Your hair could look dull and possibly come out easier. And your nails might break, 'way too often'!

Beautiful skin looks like porcelain, the stuff that expensive cups and plates are made from. Beautiful hair is strong enough to comb without fear. And beautiful nails mean that you spend less money on getting fake ones!

During sleep, the rate of beauty cell production doubles. Talk about 'beauty sleep'. Mother Nature planned this visit to your *private salon* for a reason. Next time you see your bed, just think 'free treatments' and go get them!

SLEEP BOOSTS EVERYTHING GOOD

One of the other chemicals boosted during sleep, is growth hormone. It's a little different to other hormones, in that its biggest surge happens in the first few hours *after* you drift off. The better you sleep, the bigger this surge will be.

Why does growth hormone matter? Because it boosts most of our other good chemicals. That alone is enough to recommend maxing it out. But growth hormone is no one-trick pony. He's a stunt horse who can do it all and make you look amazing!

He helps thicken your skin, which we've just seen, gets a make-over during sleep. He also rebuilds your muscle tissue, and makes your tendons and ligaments stronger (the stringy bits that hold your skeleton and muscles together).

And although that might sound un-sexy, it's not. For you to have continuous success, you need to be continuously injury-free and not be sick (and only that way can you be *anxiety-free*). Growth hormone helps with all that stuff. But there's more.

Growth hormone burns fat *while* you sleep, especially if you haven't overeaten too close to bedtime. Although your liver mainly fuels the night shift, growth hormone helps out too. Just a reminder, **the first few hours of sleep are vital**.

And even beyond those first hours, growth hormone keeps being released in little bursts. Each of these reaches out all over your body, making skin, muscles, and even your hair and nails grow properly. Feeling sleepy yet? Hold on!

SLEEP BEATS BACK THE CARB BULLY

Hey, I know by now you might be sick of technical sounding words! Don't be. Give them a chance, make them your friends, and they'll love you back forever. We know that insulin is a hormone that helps us out after eating.

When we eat carbs (or even *think* about them), we release it. Too many carbs making their way into our blood at once is dangerous. So insulin shows up to mop up. And normally, it does a good job. Especially if you've been following the book.

But if you have one bad sleep, you literally become an 'overnight failure' when it comes to dealing with excess carbs. You still pump out insulin, but it seems to lose its touch at getting carbs into muscle cells.

And of course, those ever-greedy fat cells never seem to be affected by anything! After a bad night in bed, they'll absorb all the excess carbs you let them near. No joke, **you can go from healthy to almost diabetic just by sleeping badly. And being *almost* diabetic means being *totally* better at getting fatter**.

But don't worry. There's a great cure to this temporary effect. It's called sleep! The same research has shown that as soon as you catch up with sleep, your body catches up with those naughty stray carbs. Insulin starts working properly again. Good boy.

SLEEP GIVES YOU VA VA VOOM

You know what I mean, energy, zip, spark! We all know that sleeping badly makes most of the next day really *drag*. We literally can't wait to get through it and get to bed! Sleep isn't an accident of nature, but it is a disaster to miss it.

We've seen that sleep boosts your metabolism, makes your skin glow, keeps your hair, nails and muscles in tip-top shape, and even helps you deal with carbs properly. Perhaps above all of this, it gives you energy.

I'm not talking about the stuff that we can measure in a lab. I mean the stuff that *confuses* scientists and psychologists. The stuff that we can't really explain. **We don't know everything about sleep**. At least, not yet. But we do know that it allows you to *live well*.

And by that, I mean, **giving each day your best**. Okay, this is sounding extremely wishy-washy for what's supposed to be clear advice! All I can add, is that among those who make big changes in life (i.e. you!), those who sleep best, *do* the best.

Perhaps we'll eventually find the science to back up why this happens, but for now, just take a leap of faith and believe me. Sleep helps you cope with challenges. You know, like waking up and then having a COLD bath!

HOW TO SLEEP!

I had to put the exclamation mark after that title. Of course you know how to sleep! It's built-in. But there are some things which help. Some sleep tips only work for some people, but these few work for most of us.

SLEEP ONCE A DAY

Naps are for cats! Humans sleep deepest with one long sleep.

SLEEP AT NIGHT

We need to avoid all light to sleep, and night time is dark!

SLEEP AT ROUGHLY THE SAME TIME

It doesn't have to be exact! Sleep just likes a regular pattern.

SLEEP WITH AN ALARM SET, BUT DON'T USE IT

Have one just in case, but aim to get up when you feel like it.

SLEEP WITHOUT FEELING HUNGRY OR FULL

You'll either end up in the kitchen or the bathroom!

SLEEP IS THE ONLY THING A BED IS MADE FOR

People still write that crap! A bed isn't a coffin, i.e. it's allowed more than one use!

GET THE SKINNY ON...

OMG 6 Sleep repairs all of your body and reset every major system

OMG 5 It makes sure that your metabolism burns calories properly

OMG 4 Sleep releases growth hormone which makes you lose fat

OMG 3 Growth hormone repairs muscle which keeps you healthy

OMG 2 It also makes your hair, skin and nails grow beautifully

OMG 1 Sleep helps insulin deal with excess carbs properly

OMG ! Let nothing stop you from having an amazing sleep!

THIRSTY WORK

Water. Plain, simple and free. Okay, maybe it's not always *free*. Does water really deserve its own chapter? It does. After all, we're pretty much a giant sack of the stuff! This remarkable clear liquid impacts fat loss and much more.

POWER FROM NOTHING

Water keeps you going. Not bad for something with zero calories. How can this be? For starters, if your cells aren't topped up with fluid, they don't work properly. And I'm actually talking about all cells.

Cells are like footballs. If they're not properly full (yes I *know* footballs aren't full of water!), they don't work. They literally can't fulfill their purpose. If any of your cells are dehydrated, they just shut down.

Muscle cells are no different. But where they are different, is unlike many types of cells, if you don't let them drink properly, they'll hit back hard in a very obvious way. They'll make you physically weaker.

If you give them just 3% less than they want, they'll drop your performance level by up to 30%. That's a serious splash of bad karma! And if you're feeling that much weaker, you'll hardly be able to get through your normal day.

What's more dangerous, is if you're just *slightly* dehydrated. Why? Because you might put your tiredness down to a bad sleep, bad food, or even 'just a bad hair day'! And underneath *all* that, 'Oh man, why am I *so* tired?' guesswork, it could simply be your personal drought.

When you're active during your movement sessions, you'll sweat more and lose water in each breath. After you've finished, you'll still lose water at a faster rate because you're still cooling. You can even lose water when you're *in* water.

WATER MAKES YOU GROW

When we don't have enough water, our production of growth hormone seems to drop. Not only that, but it doesn't get a boost during movement, something that's normally as predictable as guys drooling at *Angelina*.

The biology and chemistry of this aren't simple (I'm talking about growth hormone, not why guys ogle *Angie*, that *is* simple!). Dehydration stops growth hormone in its tracks. In case you've forgotten, growth hormone builds muscle, strips fat, and even improves your skin quality.

Much of our body's water supply is controlled by the **kidneys**. If you lose too much water, your brain and kidneys have a chat, and *stop* you from visiting the toilet! You save water. But if you need water in a hurry, it will come *from* the blood.

Obviously, there's a limit to what the body can do. After all, we're not connected to a fire hydrant. So, it needs a bit of help.

For the curious ones, how much water you have doesn't seem to affect the wrinkling of your skin.

That's because wrinkles start at the lowest level of the skin called the **dermis**. The dermis is always full of water, just like the water table in soil. It's damaged through too much UV (sun), too much junk (diet), and too much use, e.g. frowning (do you want to tell *Kristen* or shall I?).

HAS ANYONE SEEN MY WATER?

So, you know that having enough water keeps your muscles happy, and that they'll return the favor by not making you weak. You also know that being topped up makes sure that growth hormone gets a proper boost from movement.

The question on your parched lips is now, 'how much water do I need?'. For years, smart scientists have been designing ridiculously complicated answers to this simple question. Perhaps our obsession with water has kept them locked in the lab.

There's the public friendly '8 glasses of water per day' idea, special formulas (I told you we'd never escape them!), and theories where you constantly monitor the color of your urine at every visit to the bathroom!

But the answer is obvious. **Drink when you're thirsty.** Immediately, I can hear you screaming, 'by then it's too late!', or perhaps the intelligent sounding, 'thirst is not a good indicator of hydration'. Flapdoodle poodle!

Our body's control of its water level is outstanding. In the age of modern tech, our systems are far superior to anything that's been invented. In fact, our control of water only goes wrong during extreme situations. Like?

Like during times of constant, intense movement, in hot weather. For example, during a marathon. Even then, care must be taken to not go over the top. Runners die from drinking too much water, because they dilute chemicals that keep their heart ticking.

Back to under watering. It takes a certain kind of mind to ignore the thirst signal. One that *forces* itself to do nothing about it. And if you do keep doing that, you'll eventually run (or crawl) into trouble. So, **just pay attention to your thirst**.

To replace water, your body takes it from anywhere. Water itself is the quickest, followed by foods with lots of water in them. And actually, that's most foods. Even dry looking bread has water in it. Yes, I'm afraid there's no official reason for you to 'hydrate' bread with jam!

PLAIN SAILING

I think drinking plain water is so boring! Even so, I avoid using flavored water products. **Artificial sweeteners are bad news**. They tell your brain, 'dinner's ready', which messes with your chemistry, reducing body fat loss and increasing hunger.

You may have heard about things that make us lose water. They're called diuretics. Caffeine is one. It whispers to your kidneys, who whisper back to you by saying, 'hey, why not check out the bathroom?'!

Yet again, modern research has exaggerated this effect. Coffee and tea were always assumed to turn us into wrinkly prunes! It's really not the case. Trust your body's immaculate design, and **trust your thirst**.

I want to add one thing to this section, by talking about adding *nothing*. **Your body just wants water.** It doesn't need the minerals of *mineral water*. And actually, most of those are low in minerals! Eat food for minerals.

In terms of how clean your water is, it's smart to get the best you can find. And that's tricky. Bottled water is often up to 2 years old by the time you sip it. Sitting in dark warehouses for 100 weeks is hardly the freshness I was shown in the commercials!

Finally, drinking water with meals doesn't really stop you from overeating. But, if you have something *instead* of water, like a soft drink, you'll definitely be getting more calories (and pretty lame ones at that).

GET THE SKINNY ON . . .

OMG 6 We need water, not too much, not too little

OMG 5 If muscle cells don't drink enough, you'll be weaker

OMG 4 Weakness leads to tiredness which leads to less caloriesness!

OMG 3 Dehydration stops growth hormone from working properly

OMG 2 Your body will get water from all liquids and even solid food

OMG 1 Avoid using flavored water as sweeteners ruin appetite and fat burning

OMG ! Just listen out for thirst, and when you hear it, drink!

THE NOT SO CUTE DIMPLES

Cellulite. Apparently, it's only been around since 1968 when the word first entered our language. Strangely, if you ask most females, they'll insist that it's, 'been around forever'! This odd and confidence shattering problem affects so many girls.

What *is* cellulite? Well, for those of you who have it, you'll definitely know what it looks like. Most common on female thighs, it appears as small dimples that become especially noticeable as legs get stretched, squeezed or wobble.

Many scientists, even in 2012, can't agree about *what* cellulite is. Although most of this is due to honest scientific confusion, some of the uncertainty might be due to shady reasons. Those reasons are the *business* of cellulite.

LUMP SUMS

Cellulite is rarely researched by the medical community. Despite this, every few years, 'new' research seems to surface. Here's a great piece of advice. Never be fooled by the term **clinical studies**.

A clinical study, is a study, in a clinic. Any clinic! You could set one up in *your* bedroom. I wouldn't advise calling it 'My Bedroom Clinic' though! Perhaps something Latin like, 'Domus Research' ('House Research'). See what I mean?

206

These sneaky but entirely legal definitions lead us to believe that we're listening to scientific fact. Most clinical studies are paid for by cosmetic companies who would be better described as creators of science fiction!

The only genuine studies are called **peer-reviewed**, and they appear in science journals read by peers (the eldest geeks). And when it comes to cellulite, there are far less studies than you've been lead to believe.

So, what do we *really* know? First off is the annoying biggie. Genetics. Although up to 80% of women get cellulite, it varies in how bad it looks, and most of that is no one's fault. I've got to ask, why didn't you pick the right parents?

The second thing we know, is that it's extremely rare in men. This is a big clue. Guys have tougher skins. When some men lose testosterone (a hormone) they start to get cellulite. Testosterone thickens the skin. The plot thickens too!

Thirdly, we've noticed that as most women age, cellulite appears to get worse. As most people age, they've probably spent more time in the sun, more time on a bad diet, and more time being generally unhealthy. Clues, clues, clues.

When we put all these factors together, it seems that **cellulite is small pockets of unevenly spaced out fat, just below the skin**. Cause? Either fat isn't being laid down evenly, or some of it is un-attaching itself while other bits cling on.

If it's about fat being put down unevenly, what could be causing that? We have fat cells all over. *Where* these fat cells set-up camp, gets decided as you are decided. That means, the minute you were 'hatched', for want of a cheekier word!

Although you can't choose *where* fat cells are, it doesn't mean those cells have to *be* fat. Fat cells can be stuffed full of fat, or they can be like empty grocery bags. This means that even if you've got lots of fat cells, you're not automatically destined to become the world see-saw champion!

But, if you choose to pile on the pudge, fat cells happily swell, absorbing any junk you chuck at them. Eventually, even *they* get full. If you push the little fatties further, they become big fatties, and then, BANG, they burst in half. Yes, they double! That's a 2-for-1 that nobody bargains for.

It could be that when *that* happens, we get the stuff we call, cellulite. Fat cells reaching their limits (limits personal to you), some splitting, and then the laying down of more cells in random places. **A massive cellular explosion and relocation under the surface**.

This only happens if you allow yourself to get fat. How fat? Hard to say. In some people, in some areas of the body, it happens easy. Definitely, if you develop more fat cells, you'll raise your potential for total fatness. Not good!

To avoid this, **stay slim while you're still young**. That's possibly all the way until reaching 21. After that point, it becomes much harder for fat cells to split. Although, for those of you who want to break fat cell high scores, it's not impossible!

SKINNY GIRL CELLULITE

Some of you might be reading this and thinking, 'I know girls who aren't fat, but *still* have cellulite, what about them?'. And you'd have a point. Cellulite is generally less common in skinny people, but it can exist. Why?

It could be what you've read, combined with another problem. The *quality* of your skin. The skin is our biggest organ and an outside reflection of what's going on inside. And the inside's always complicated!

Going back to what we know about men and cellulite, it seems that even when men get fat, they still rarely get cellulite. Men's skin is usually thicker than women's. This is because they have slightly more **collagen** and **elastin**.

These are the bricks and cement of skin, and they literally hold it together. If you build a strong wall, you won't know what's going on behind it. Build a more fragile wall, or damage the one you have, and it's a different story.

Thicker skin appears smoother, no matter what's happening under the surface. Men could have similar amounts of fat cells, and cells bursting at the seams, but because their skin is tougher, you wouldn't know. *So* not fair!

HOW TO GET EVEN

Okay, you're fed up reading about men's genetic luck! You want to know if there's anything you can do to get rid of cellulite.

There is. You've met all these ideas before, but now you might see them in a different light.

BUMPS IN THE NIGHT

Yep, as boring as it sounds, a good sleep will help your thighs. It's because sleep is the thing that produces a huge surge of growth hormone. Growth hormone definitely thickens the skin, which makes it smoother, and less likely to let little bumps show through.

IT TAKES AGES

Even if you ignore how excess carbs make you fat, it eventually becomes hard to ignore what they do to your skin. Too many carbs will create **Advanced Glycation End Products**, abbreviated to *AGES*. I know, it actually shortens to *AGEP*. Hey, let the geeks feel naughty!

What are AGES? They're proteins that have got damaged by excess levels of carbs clinging to them. Collagen and elastin, your skin's bricks and cement, are proteins whose structure is easily damaged this way. As you can imagine, it's hard to build a quality wall (skin) with broken bricks.

Damage from AGES affects most of the body. In skin, they cause weakening and wrinkling, which makes cellulite worse, or more likely. They even affect our heart and arteries. There could be nutrients in plants that help protect against this, but it's tricky to research.

The way to combat AGES is to eat a diet with a smart level of carbs. In particular, it's really important to avoid man-made sugars (including those which end in '...ose'). They attack collagen and elastin quickest, making your skin older than your birth certificate suggests.

If you've been eating badly for a while, changing to lower carbs will bring about really visible changes. In 6 weeks, you will have made 2 to 3 lots of entirely new, better-fed skin, and it will look *much* healthier. Do it for a year, and you could turn back the clock 10 years* (*Individual results may vary, i.e. if you're 12, I can't make you look 2 again!).

USE THE IRON TO SMOOTH THINGS OVER

Doing weights could help cellulite disappear (or not appear). Pumping iron not only increases growth hormone, which thickens skin, but it also can forcefully increase the flow of blood in one area. And that's a great thing.

All movement shifts the blood around, but when you just concentrate on moving one area, blood is *really* squeezed around. If you do weights movements for your thighs, your muscles sneak blood into the smallest nooks and crannies.

Some research *suggests* that cellulite's uneven appearance could be due to some cells not getting a decent flow of blood and nutrients. This may or may not turn out to be correct. But, it definitely does no harm to improve blood flow.

So, keep doing your general movement, but also make sure that you do weights at least 3 times per month, and include a movement for your thighs. When you think about it, that probably takes just 30 minutes per month. Definitely worth it.

DRAIN HARDER

In a few sections, *Skinny Dipping* and *Party Tricks With Balloons*, we met something called the lymphatic system. It's our second bloodstream, containing stuff including proteins and fats, and white blood cells which help kill off diseases.

As we just read, some research suggests that cellulite might be areas with poor circulation. Boosting blood flow is one way to improve this, but it might be useful to drain our lymphatic system. I say drain, which means to shift the fluid *around*.

And to do that, body brushing while *skinny dipping* could help. Remember, it needs light pressure, and you must always brush *towards* the heart. Thankfully, in a bath, you can just about reach the main area of cellulite, the thighs.

The only other way to increase the flow of the lymphatic system, is to breathe deeply. Often, experts mention things like jogging as helping it. They work, but not strictly to do with the jogging itself. It's mainly from the tag-along increase in breathing.

When we take a deep breath in, the pressure inside us builds up, and it forces lots of lymphatic fluid to flush around the system. Blowing up balloons is great, because it gets us into a pattern of regular and deep breathing.

Although blowing up balloons heavily works on the blowing-out muscles (which flatten your tummy), we naturally take deep breaths in too. Deep breathing is also great for general health and growth hormone release, so keep those balloons floating!

Yes, just that. The beginning of the chapter talked about fat cells filling up, but it needs a quick reminder. **The greatest thing you can do to reduce cellulite, or avoid it, is to make sure you're the right size.** And that definitely means not being too fat.

I can't give you an exact body weight, or size for your thighs. The answer is hidden deep in your genetic code. I can say, if you **get skinnier**, you'll have reduced the size of individual fat cells, and that will improve your skin's structure.

THE TRUTH ABOUT CELLULITE 'CURES'

They don't work. What a way to start a paragraph. I just didn't want to waste your time. Your time would be much better spent moving, eating better and even doing nothing (sleeping). The beauty industry squats somewhere between the food and drug industry.

Because of that, it usually escapes the regulations that occur on either side. As I mentioned before, clinical trials mean very little. Most creams cannot get down into the dermis, which is your deepest layer of skin. Some fat cells are even deeper still.

Even if you see the words, 'improves the appearance of', take a step back and read the sentence again. It means, 'we can't fix it, but we'll hide it for a few hours'. Fine if you're heading out to party, but realize that cellulite won't truly be leaving town.

Liposuction is not a good solution. It can remove large numbers of fat cells, but it can also produce heavy scarring. There's no way to predict how your skin, or entire body, will respond to having surgery. Be kind to you. Do other stuff.

GET THE SKINNY ON...

OMG 6 Cellulite is probably too many or too large fat cells for your skin

OMG 5 The first strategy must be to reduce your body fat in general

OMG 4 If you're under 21, stay skinny to prevent fat cells doubling

OMG 3 Sleep deep to boost growth hormone which makes skin stronger

OMG 2 Keep carbs low as high levels will damage skin's structure

OMG 1 Body brush in the bath to boost lymphatic circulation

OMG ! Use all of the tips and see what happens in 2 to 3 weeks!

GREEN WITH ENVY

Although coffee is brilliant for the morning, you can't just keep drinking cup after cup throughout the day. Too much of anything tends to not be good for you. And coffee, including the caffeine it contains, also gets bad if you have too much.

Coffee boosts your central nervous system, so chugging it all the time could make you overly wired. At worst, it might make your heart beat out of rhythm. That's scary to feel and can even be dangerous.

And for some people, having endless caffeine reduces its effect. This is simply the body trying to protect itself from being over-stimulated. After it does this, it takes way more caffeine than before to get the same boost.

To avoid this, it's best to drink your main source of caffeine once per day, and ideally, soon after waking up. This way, you get all the benefits and none of the problems. Eventually though, caffeine wears itself out.

That takes about 6 hours. After that, we're still left with a big chunk of the day. Luckily, nature has given us another secret potion! **Green tea**. It does have some caffeine, but not enough for chaos. And it contains other good stuff.

Green tea leaves are from the same family as normal tea, but they haven't been allowed to react with the air for as long. Because of this freshness, green tea contains high amounts of something called **Epigallocatechin Gallate**. Memorize that.

Surely you didn't believe me! EGCG, for short, is a potent little beast. It does up to three amazing things all at once. Because green tea is cheap and easy to get, it would be crazy to not put it in your arsenal against fat.

THE GREEN TEA SCARECROW

Green tea seems to lower appetite, and that's fab. This doesn't mean that you stop looking forward to food completely! It just places appetite where it's supposed to be. Not too high and not too low. Just *right*.

It does this by raising a chemical called nor-epinephrine (also known as nor-adrenaline). This chemical is released when your body thinks that it's being threatened (e.g. by a dinosaur, co-worker, teacher) And because of that, **green tea can reduce appetite**.

Digestion takes a bit of energy and a lot of blood supply. If your brain thinks you're about to get into a fight, it needs you to have oxygen where it's needed. That's your heart and your muscles. Appetite dampens down.

THE GREEN TEA FURNACE

The chemical we just talked about, nor-epinephrine, reduces digestion. But the body isn't stupid, and it realizes that if you're in trouble, and if you've stopped processing food in your stomach, you'll need to get energy from somewhere eventually.

Ta da! Green tea acts like the equally green *Shrek*, breaking *Princess Fiona* out of her tower. In our analogy, the Princess represents previously locked-up body fat! Apologies, your highness. **Green tea helps you 'rescue' stored fat energy, and use it.**

THE GREEN TEA SHEEP DOG

Green tea's chemicals also help you deal with all those excess carbs after a meal. It does this by making your muscles more able to absorb them. This means that any leftover carbs are less likely to end up inside fat cells.

It does this by making your insulin work better. Yet *again*, I remind you of how important it is to do that. Insulin is a shepherd whose job involves taking nutrients out of the blood, and getting them into cells.

Its main job description is to get carbs into muscles. But it also has a small but important role with *other* nutrients. I call this its *sheep dog role* (instead of the *shepherd role*, which is finding a space for the flock of excess carbs).

The green tea sheep dog helps you get nutrients like *protein*, *vitamins* and *minerals* into muscle cells, and even into your organs. This is great if you're losing body fat, as it makes sure that your calorie burning muscles stay healthy.

Dieting causes some people to lose lots of muscle weight. For many reasons, losing muscle is a bad thing. It's crazy, but this

217

little drink of green tea helps insulin work, which in turn helps muscles keep strong. Result!

WE WORK GREAT TOGETHER

Green tea works best when you *combine* it with other healthy things. For example, everything you read in this book! By itself, it seems to increase calorie loss by about 50 to 100 per day. But of course, calories aren't the whole story.

When it's combined with extra movement and better food choices, it's possible that the effect of green tea is much more powerful. This is called **synergy**. It's where individual changes somehow are worth more *together*, i.e. it's a fancy way of saying that $1 + 1 + 1 = 4$.

WHEN AND HOW TO DRINK GREEN TEA

We're all different, but research suggests that green tea really starts to have an effect when you drink about 2 to 4 cups per day. That's 16 to 32 ounces (about 500ml to 1000ml). I know, that sounds like a scary amount of liquid!

There are green tea supplements (like capsules and tablets). I don't recommend them. Why? Well, you'll rattle loudly! Seriously, whenever possible, a natural source is usually the purest and safest. Stick to the liquid.

Hot tea is hard to drink. In fact, you might hate the taste of green tea whatever its temperature! You could let it cool down completely, and use it as a water substitute throughout the day, or around the time of your movement sessions.

Remember, it's the special chemicals we want, and therefore **don't add sugar or milk to your green tea**. If you do, you'll cancel out the fat burning effects. It's better to have no green tea, than a green tea happy frappe chappy mocha choca latte!

Most modern store brands are good quality. Perhaps still best, are the loose tea leaves that you can buy from a Chinese medicine store. The main thing is that you let the tea (or tea bag) sit in the hot water for about 3 to 5 minutes.

If you drink green tea with your meals, you might want to drink it at the end. Although green tea before boosts helpful chemicals quickly and fills you up, there's no point in reducing how nice a meal *feels*.

The caffeine content of green tea, in the amounts I've suggested, is low enough to not cause a problem in most people. As I always keep saying, we're all different, and if you find adding it makes you less sleepy at night, cut back a cup.

GET THE SKINNY ON...

OMG 6 Green tea has EGCG, a chemical that boosts neurotransmitters

OMG 5 These will reduce your appetite slightly

OMG 4 They also increase body fat burning between meals

OMG 3 Green tea makes insulin better at absorbing excess carbs

OMG 2 Drink 2 to 4 cups per day (16 to 32 ounces / 500 to 1000ml)

OMG 1 Don't add milk or sugar if possible

OMG ! Go get some green tea and make 'em green with envy!

HYPE AND TYPE

Most of us are happy to believe what we read. If it's in black and white, *it must be true*. Official looking type looks more factual than old fashioned handwriting. But this habit of seeing and believing can be dangerous for your health.

This section is a hodgepodge of things you need to know when you venture out into...the grocery store! It can be a confusing place, and sometimes, it's full of lies. **You need to be smart to beat the business of hype and type**, but it *can* be done.

IS IT A GIFT OR A PACKAGE?

Packaging. Tells. Lies. It's not there to help you. It's there to sell product. The food business is huge, and to stand out, companies have to do whatever they can to distract you from buying a different brand. How would you do it?

Years ago, they just made claims about their product's taste. Although taste is personal, marketing it is still honest. But today, companies know that we don't just buy food for its taste, or even how it looks. We link food to our body.

When I say body, I mean two different aspects. We think about how a food affects *our outsides* and how a food affects *our insides*. Bright packaging and nice taste have limits, but there is no limit to our imaginations, our worries and our hopes.

From time to time, we all have worries. It might be our weight, our skin, or perhaps just how well we feel. So we also have hopes of being the weight we want, having great skin, and feeling super healthy. I mean, who *wouldn't* want all that?

We carry these thoughts around, looking for answers. Whether you're in a store, watching TV, or just out walking, our brain is scanning for ways to have its worries reduced or our hopes satisfied. Food companies *depend* on this.

And they use it to design and market food products that tick all your boxes. In theory, governments have departments to make sure that companies can't tell us lies. That's a tough job, and well, somebody's got to do it badly!

Beginning in the 1980s, the foods on our shelves started changing. They became good for your heart, good for your weight, low in calories, low in fat and more recently they've being getting high. Getting high *in nutrients*, come on!

As our obsession with health and looking good grows, so does the obsession of companies who want to make money from it. The trouble is, companies have got greedy. And now, almost every product in our stores has 'healthy' slapped on it!

It's true that no food deserves to be called 'unhealthy', unless it's all you eat or drink. But, it's also fair to say that not all foods can be thought of *as* 'healthy', i.e. just eating *more* of it makes you *more* healthy.

As soon as the sharks started to call their foods 'healthy', the little fish had to do the same, or risk having their customers switch brands. The yogurt, cereal and drinks industries started the trend, and they're certainly not going to remove those magic 7 letters.

There are a few ways that food companies (and stores) use *hype and type*. Let's take a look at some of the main ones. Once you're aware of them, you'll be able to stride through the grocery store with a smart spring in your step.

POISON FROG FOOD

Organic is still such a cool buzz word. Organic food guarantees that it won't contain any artificial chemicals. And that's great, because who knows what certain chemicals could do in the long-term. But 'organic' can't guarantee that a food is healthy.

Deep in the Amazon rain forest, there are frogs that have skin that's deadly to touch. Some of these are more poisonous than *anything* we can make in a chemistry lab. I mean, even today, we *still* can't out-poison them. But guess what, they are organic!

Don't you just love extreme frog analogies! Look, if I've *decided* on a food, and there's a choice of two versions, organic or not, I'll go organic. But I know that when it comes to certain foods, organic means nothing more than a word that uses all your *Scrabble* tiles!

Food companies use 'organic' to sell us stuff that we might normally walk past. If you're health conscious, the words 'organic pizza' instantly sound less naughty than just 'pizza'. I literally just licked my lips after writing that sentence!

Using organic is like laying down all 7 letters in *Scrabble*, you get a bonus. But it's not the game won. Governments try to restrict food companies talking up health claims, but they can't stop them shouting 'organic' from the grocery store rooftops.

And they can't stop us thinking, organic *means* healthy. So, the next time you see *organic* **chocolate**, *organic* **ice cream**, *organic* **pizza**, or *organic* **anything**, delete the word organic, and *then* make your decision about whether it feels right to eat.

In the future, I hope that all our food is organic. Just like it used to be. And if it becomes like that again, we'll all be able to forget anything other than whether a food is *healthy to start with*. Until then, be smart. **Mentally delete 'organic',** *then* **choose**.

PANDA AND POTTER FOOD

Pandas eat 30 pounds of bamboo per day. Per day! Dude, read the section on plate size! For years, we didn't know why. Scientists recently discovered that somewhere down the line, something convinced Pandas that's all they could eat. Weird.

We know that it's altered their body, and now, bamboo is pretty much all they can eat. The problem with bamboo, is that it's a rubbish food! It has hardly any nutrients, and that's exactly why Pandas need to eat so much of it.

Why am I talking about Pandas? Well, they're furry and cuddly and...Right, Pandas are an example that us fuzz-free types can learn from. Many of our foods claim to be 'high in' something good, when that's not really true at all. Let's go human now.

Popcorn. If you squint hard enough, you could say that it contains calcium. We all love calcium, it's the stuff that makes our bones strong. Do you know how much popcorn you'd need to eat in order to get a decent chunk of calcium?

You'd have to munch your way through all 8 *Harry Potter* movies (*including* number 5)! Or you could watch 1, 2 and 3 (fun), step out into the foyer, swig a glass of milk, and go home with plenty calcium and zero *Potter* regret!

The point is, no one must be forced to watch *The Order of the Phoenix!* Seriously, companies often tell us that their foods are 'high in' something, *when they're not*. Common highs are 'high in fiber' or 'high in xxx', where xxx is a mega nutrient.

Take bread. In some countries, to be called 'high fiber', a food has to have more than 3 grams of fiber per serving. It's a useful amount, 3 grams. But the problem is, **governments can't force companies to fix what a serving size (portion) means**.

One company might make bread with '3 grams of fiber per serving', and that serving size might be *a slice*. Another company might also have '3 grams of fiber per serving', but their serving might need to be *4 slices*. Why the little sneaks!

These *Panda and Potter* principles are useful throughout most grocery store visits. Serving sizes often need to be so huge just to get a tiny amount of the 'high in' healthy stuff that we originally signed up for!

Overall, **these tricks make us buy food that we don't really need**. These foods promise to make us *healthy*, but they usually just make us *eat too much*. And often, it's *carbs* who we really end up over scoffing.

SOLE FOOD

So many foods claim to be 'healthy' because they contain the hot new nutrient kid on the block. If you walk *around* the block, and then analyze the mud on the sole of your shoes, you'll find some kind of mega nutrient. I'm serious! Get a microscope.

But obviously, there's no money to be made from companies getting you to lick your soles! If you did try it, you'd have to lick a lot of mud to get a tiny amount of special nutrients. And at the same time, you'd probably get lots of bad stuff.

Sounds extreme, but it's pretty much how many foods are. Promoted as being 'healthy', they actually have *few* good nutrients and *lots* of bad stuff. And that's the true naughty nature of these foods: low nutritional bang for your buck.

Here's a great example. Fruit juice that doesn't contain virtually any fruit juice! There are many of these on the market. I'm certainly not claiming that fruit juice is healthy itself, but if I bought some, I'd want some fruit juice in it!

In the case of that product, you would find artificial flavors, artificial colorings, artificial sweeteners, artificial preservatives, and lots of man-made sugar. And yet you could have bought *for* its fruit juice, which is usually around just 10% of it!

Some products jump on whatever the most recent media bandwagon might be. Take **lycopene**, a plant chemical plentiful in

225

tomatoes that can reduce ageing. When news hit town about its benefits, every bottle of ketchup suddenly became 'healthy'.

Ketchup does contain lycopene, but it's the tomatoes that make it like that. Not the tons of added sugar in the ketchup, or the flavorings, or the preservatives. And even in the amounts that people use ketchup, it's not easy to get a meaningful amount.

It's also worth saying that some companies talk-up nutrients because of recent research discoveries, when in fact, the discovery isn't *really* a discovery. I mean, the importance of the research itself might have been exaggerated.

You were getting on well in your life without lycopene, but as soon as you knew about it, you 'had' to have it! You had to get the extra carbs too. Lycopene is just one of thousands, if not millions of plant chemicals around. Panic over.

Like the *Panda and Potter* principles, *Sole Food* is something to watch out for. Don't be swayed by claims of something being 'healthy'. The healthiest foods don't need to SHOUT!!! about it. Foods that do shout, often (*hide*) lots of unhealthy stuff too.

HAPPY CLAPPY FOOD

This is the very latest in naughty food. Products that claim you'll *feel* good if you have them. Yogurt companies are probably the best example around. Let me get this straight, many yogurts are excellent foods. Can you hear the 'but' tiptoeing?

But, some yogurt companies are just never satisfied! They've managed to sell us 'fat-free' yogurts (high carb), 'high-in calcium'

226

yogurts (need to eat a bucket's worth), and 'low lactose' yogurts (they never contained much lactose in the first place).

They've now moved on much further. They've invented 'feel better' yogurts. *Feel* better? Surely that's a very personal thing, how you feel. These guys are smart. They learned from the cosmetic industries. They did 'trials'.

Strictly speaking, they don't claim 'clinical trials', but they do the next best thing. They have slogans like, '8 out of 10 women felt a zillion times better after two weeks'. Everyone wants to be part of the 'in' crowd.

Companies know that they can't directly claim their product makes you feel better or more beautiful. But they can tell you about others who said it did *exactly* that! It's an example of 'we didn't say that, she did'. And boy does it work!

All you need is a hungry and poor group of random people to try your food, and then fill out a survey. If the group says it made them feel good, you can tell customers about it. Two problems. The people aren't random, and there's not enough of them.

Most people who fill in surveys, are random. But food researchers don't like this street corner approach. They like to advertise, find people, look after them well, and pay them. If you do that for strangers, they'll generally be nice back!

Food (and cosmetic) companies keep surveys small. This means under a 1000 or even a 100 sometimes. Bigger groups are just *too* tricky to schmooze! BTW, if 75% of people liked something, 25% didn't. Even *after* you paid and waited on them!

The point is, we often buy these foods based on shaky claims, and assume that if we have them, we'll 'feel better' too. These foods usually are laced with tons of sugar, and **once we've started buying them, we keep buying them out of sheer habit.**

All of the foods types we've mentioned, *rely* on **hype and type**. If we're not careful, we can easily end up believing their claims, and eat stuff that we don't really *need*. **Whenever you see the word 'healthy' written on something, assume that it's unhealthy, and let it prove its innocence *after* close inspection.**

GET THE SKINNY ON . . .

OMG 6 Food packaging is designed to sell the product

OMG 5 Organic food is chemical-free but still doesn't guarantee health

OMG 4 Foods 'high in' something good may need big portions to get it

OMG 3 That may make you overeat calories, carbs, or both

OMG 2 Don't be fooled into buying nutrients you weren't looking for

OMG 1 Don't shop when you're hungry, or hype and type might GET!!! you

OMG ! Be wary of any foodstuff that's labeled 'healthy'!

CROP ROTATION

When it comes to fruits and vegetables, it's wise to choose as many different ones as possible. This advice is something that applies to all humans, whether they're dieting or have never even uttered the 'D' word.

As smart as science is, it doesn't know everything yet. In the last 10 years, we've discovered the 'miracles' of blueberries, and then pomegranate, and then goji berries, and then acai berries, and so the list goes on.

Each new discovery, while adding to our knowledge, is also like nature saying, 'you don't know everything'. And until we do (if ever), it's smart to try different fruits and vegetables. **Rotate your crops!**

People often talk about the Amazon rainforest as being an *Aladdin's Cave* of plants, but so what? Most of us haven't even explored 10% of what's in our grocery store caves! We tend to be creatures of habit.

A study once found that people with super low rates of cancer also had the highest variety of foods in their diet. In fact, these walking temples had over 50 different food types per week. This is an interesting study, even if you just want to lose fat.

Researchers also found that good variety walks hand in hand with good legs. So, is being skinny due to having a big mix of mega nutrients? Or from avoiding too much of one naughty food? Who knows. But there's a secret to be had.

There may be things in plants that are super useful in fat loss. And also, there may be things in some plants that make it more difficult. Until our scientific knowledge catches up, **it's smart to have variety**.

The cool thing about switching around your fresh stuff, is that it helps you forget that you're 'on a diet'. It's a crucial taste of freedom. **One guaranteed way that diets stop, is when the person on them gets bored**.

Now I'm not pretending that switching from apples to peaches is exciting, or that eating red peppers instead of green gets the pulse racing, but it might help you avoid boredom. What is exciting, is sticking to your plan and getting those OMGs!

GET THE SKINNY ON...

OMG 6 Vegetables and fruits contain healthy nutrients

OMG 5 Some of these haven't been discovered or named yet

OMG 4 Fruit and veg may contain things that speed fat loss

OMG 3 They may also contain things that block fat loss

OMG 2 Research shows that people who mix it up are skinniest

OMG 1 Variety in your fruit and veg may help prevent diet boredom

OMG ! Eat every fruit and vegetable available at least once!

DITCH DOUBLE DIGIT DISKS

Quite a tongue twister. Talking of tongues, one of the best ways to eat smarter, is to use smaller plates. I'm actually not asking you to eat from a saucer here! I'm suggesting going back to the plate sizes used when people were much skinnier.

In simple terms, **any double digit plate size is asking for food trouble**. That means a 10 inch plate isn't smart. Your upper limit for a plate must really be about 9 inches (about 23 centimeters). Obviously, restaurants let you choose food mainly and not plates!

But for meals at home, use a smaller plate. Buy one if you have to. The temptation with a bigger plate is to simply eat everything on it. There's all kinds of psychology going on with that, and it's hard to block out. **Buy a smaller plate!**

There's a place called *Okinawa*. It's a small group of islands near Japan. The people who live there often reach 100, and they're always skinny and healthy. They have a saying. It's, 'hara hachi bu'. Apparently *Confucius* said it. Confused?

I was until *Google Translate* arrived! It means, 'Eat until you're eight tenths full'. That doesn't mean eat 80% of *any* plate, because your plate could be the size of a Panda's! The Okinawan's use smaller plates, and so can you. *Domo arigato!*

GET THE SKINNY ON...

OMG 6 We eat with our eyes, not with our stomachs

OMG 5 If there's space on your plate you'll fill it and fill up

OMG 4 Nine inch plates are big enough and may stop you overeating

OMG 3 Picking smaller cups might also help

OMG 2 Social pressures create guilt about leaving food uneaten

OMG 1 Reduce this with small plates at home and small portions when out

OMG ! Use small plates even if that means baby or animal ones!

WHO'S COUNTING?

In 1824, a French scientist, tucked away in a secret lab in the middle of Europe, discovered your worst nightmare. Scarier than *Frankenstein* and able to appear in daylight (unlike *Robert Pattinson*) he discovered, THE CALORIE!

If this was *Harry Potter*, dietary fat would be a *Death Eater* and the calorie would be *Lord Voldemort!* Calories are evil. They're everywhere. And they must be destroyed. Is that true, does the calorie really *deserve* its bad reputation?

First of all, let me explain what a **calorie** is. A calorie is the energy it takes to heat up about 2 pounds of water by about 2 degrees Fahrenheit. Yes that's right, calories are all about heating up a big kettle!

Years ago, scientists took chunks of various foods, put them in a large device, and 'burned' them. The more it heated up the water, the more energy it had in it. Scientists called this energy, calories (from *calor*, the Latin for *heat*).

Bizarrely, if you drink very cold water, your body spends a tiny amount of energy in heating it up to body temperature. The effect is small, so you can cancel that journey to your local swimming pool right now!

Today, they don't set foods on fire, but analyze them chemically instead. Anyways, is any of this calorie stuff important? Nope. Technically, humans must 'obey the laws of physics', which calories are part of. Obey sounds like *should* in another coat!

Physics states that energy (calories) can't be created or destroyed. They say that energy just changes into different forms. This is supposed to mean that by controlling calories, we can make exact predictions about whether we'll be fat.

This could be true if our body only paid attention to physics. But it doesn't. We *obey* other subjects like biology, chemistry and bio-chemistry. Psychology too. Even physics uber geek *Einstein* admitted that he didn't know everything.

If you look at diets where the main target is simply to reduce calories, the long-term success is very low. **Our body is much smarter than dealing with numbers**. We have hormones, genes, and a massive variety of thought patterns.

With all of this combined, it's crazy to try and *just* look at calories. Even if watching calories could make you skinny, it couldn't help you control how generally healthy you were, and how healthy you looked. Want proof?

People all over our globe live on very different amounts of calories, from 1000 to 5000. And they're all skinny. How can this be? Mainly because their diets are *traditional*, i.e. many thousands of years old.

They eat natural food, the stuff they've always eaten. When they get introduced to western foods, i.e. foods changed by man, they get fat or ill or both. Without doubt, this always happens when high carb foods ride into town.

Counting calories is like whipping a horse to make it go where you want. It's much better to make friends with a nice horse, and forget the whip. That nice horse is *natural food*. And it's something that won't let you down, if you treat it well.

Counting calories is boring, and it definitely gives you a sense of anxiety. Boredom and anxiety are two feelings that you don't want for life! That's why I generally avoid talking about calories.

I wrote about them because many get scared without having an **_exact_** calorie target. And I'm well aware of formulas, diets and devices which claim to work this out. They can't. And I won't make up an answer for you.

Once you truly *get* this book, you'll be able to burn and pick smarter calories almost subconsciously. Avoiding calories themselves isn't necessary. They come from the time of *Frankenstein*, and it's a monster that you can put to bed right now!

GET THE SKINNY ON...

OMG 6 Calories are a very basic measure of heat energy in food

OMG 5 Calories from different places act differently in your body

OMG 4 Working out your daily calorie needs is an impossible task

OMG 3 Calorie formulas therefore give you a false sense of certainty

OMG 2 Good health is made from nutrients, not a number of calories

OMG 1 People with high and low calorie diets can be equally skinny

OMG ! Forget counting calories and count OMGs!

RECIPE FOR DISASTER

Stew d'OMG

(Serves no one)

Ingredients

3 Well-known diet books

1 quart of water

Brown food dye

Craft glue

Instructions

Take the diet books, and finely chop them into small pieces

Boil them in a quart of water until they really bubble

Add a dash of brown food dye, and stir for another 15 minutes

Turn off the heat, let the pan cool and add 5 spoons of craft glue

Put your life on hold for 60 minutes, and stir the mix

Remove from pan, and carefully form the mess into a ball shape

Let the shape harden overnight

Et voila

Get the ball, take a few steps back, and kick it into space!

For those who have read diet or health books before, you might still be skimming through and thinking, 'okay, where are the recipes?'. Hey, I forgot to put them in. Of course I didn't. I deliberately didn't put them in!

Recipes have no place in *Six Weeks To OMG*. Hopefully by now you've got some **confidence to pick your own foods**. Stick to half a plate of protein and keep your total daily carbs down. Avoid *the fast and the furious*. I'm summarizing, but you get it.

The only kind of book that deserves to have recipes, is a *recipe* book! Seriously. They teach people how to cook tasty new dishes. And that *improves* our relationship with food. **Diet books with recipes *damage* our relationship with food**.

Why? Because we subconsciously assume that missing foods *might* be 'bad'. Rubbish! Just because an author didn't fit them in their diet book doesn't make them a banned food. It just means that they're saving paper or electronic ink!

Diet recipes reduce true confidence. Recipes are great when you can see them, scary when you can't. You need a confidence that works in any social situation, not just at home. And if you can't cook diet recipes, that *really* dents the ego!

Do you know why recipes are always stuck at the end of a book? To make you feel okay. Recipes are there to explain what the rest of the writing couldn't! **It's much better if you understand stuff and choose food yourself.**

Recipes are also similar to what the author likes. French writers encourage French food, meat-eaters recommend just flesh, and vegetarians push plants etc. Good ideas work with endless food choices.

I don't care if you're 8 or 80. You're old enough to *not* have foods picked for you! Use the knowledge you've picked up in this book to make your own recipes.

GET THE SKINNY ON . . .

OMG 6 Recipes in diet books make absent foods seem naughty

OMG 5 Recipes in diet books reduce your confidence to choose

OMG 4 Recipes in diet books teach you to forget basic principles

OMG 3 Recipes in diet books are influenced by a writer's taste buds

OMG 2 Recipes in diet books can't last a lifetime

OMG 1 Recipes in diet books never turn out as they say

OMG ! You're an expert now so start to pick foods yourself!

AFTER SIX COMES SEVEN

So, it's about that time. You've pretty much reached the end. Perhaps you're reading the whole thing before you start. If that's the case, this section is a glimpse into your future. So many people ask, 'what do I do after I finish?'.

It depends. If you're not close to the body you had in mind when you started, you might want to keep using every technique until you get closer. You could use it all, or just use the bits that really work for *you*.

But if you *have* got to the point where you can look in the mirror and feel proud, then what? Your success will mean that most of your body's biological and chemical systems will have been really improved. They will have become efficient.

Efficient? It's a fancy way of saying that your body works well with less effort, i.e. it's easier to *stay* skinny. Even so, there are a few wonderful ideas that are practical, and always **worth it**. Here are, the seven wonders of the diet world.

1 – NEVER EAT WITHOUT MOVING FIRST

I'm not directly saying *skip breakfast*. But, **never eat first thing or at any time without doing some moving before**. This is without doubt, the best piece of advice you could ever follow when it comes to staying skinny and keeping healthy.

It's completely unnatural to eat without moving first. You can't get food in nature without moving! Our modern lifestyles maybe up to 200 years old, but our genes are over 2,000,000 years old. We must, must, must, get a wriggle on!

The ideal minimum for life is to move for 15 minutes before considering food. It's even better if you move for 15 and wait for 15. This is the *hunt and wait* idea you saw earlier in the book. Hunt down to the store, come back, and wait a bit!

15 minutes of moving changes your whole body chemistry, and giving it nothing for 15 minutes after really forces all the positive changes you could ever hope for. Truly, if you take just one point from the whole book, make it this!

It's not just about burning calories. The movement makes sure that your body becomes much better at absorbing and dealing with the food you give it. The time gap after moving boosts hormones, enzymes, and all good chemicals.

Movement does not work after meals. It just stops your digestion, ruins the nice happy feeling after a good meal, and crucially, it boosts none of the enzymes or hormones that help your body process food. Do it before, or don't bother!

So if you ever eat again, **move before you munch!** Does that look impractical or make you say, 'no way' in your head? 15 minutes is nothing. It's just 900 seconds of moving. Reading this paragraph already took you 20 seconds!

And then before your next meal, add in another bit of movement before you eat. 900 seconds, come on! Finally in the evening,

241

same again. Remember, even a walk home counts as part of this. Love your body. **Treat before you eat**.

If you're eating three times per day, you'll do three lots of moving and waiting. The most practical form of movement is to just have a quick walk. It takes no 'setting up time' and has the fewest excuses. Just move it!

Obviously these short periods aren't meant for heading out to the gym. That would be nuts. In fact, I wouldn't do anything that makes you feel like you're working out. It's not about that. Just simple, non-intense, moving around of some kind.

2 – EAT MEALS

In other words, **don't do snacks**. There is just no point in eating 6 times per day. You'll end up in the toilet all day, see the dentist more often, and you'll be fatter! Who cares if eating three times a day seems old fashioned, it works.

Eating meals is social, gives you a satisfied 'high' feeling, and makes your body's fuel gauge do its job properly. Snacks block your body from dipping into your own fat stores for energy, and that's no good. Eat meals. Enough said!

3 – STEP UP TO THE PLATE WITH PROTEIN

I'm not going to bombard you with science again. Just remember, **you're half protein and so is your ideal plate**. We lose our protein every day, and it's got to be replaced from protein in the diet. Your body needs protein above all other foods.

Because of this extreme need, your brain always looks out for it. And once you give it enough, it can relax. I mean, protein *calms* your appetite down. If you can satisfy your appetite in this natural way, you will stay skinny permanently.

The simplest way to do this? Pick a source of protein for every meal, something that's *mostly* protein, and fill half of your plate with that. Get that right, and everything else will gradually shift into place. It's that important.

Don't count the calories of your protein, or even the amount of fat in it. Watch out for carbs, especially the hidden ones in innocent looking sauces and gravies. There are healthy alternatives. **Your protein is supposed to be protein**.

4 – EAT A RAINBOW

One day, this book might seem out of date compared to what scientists go onto discover. But one thing will *never* change. And that's fruits and vegetables. We need them. They are nature's secret colorful potions.

It might sound simplistic, but getting a variety of colors into your diet is one of the easiest ways to get a variety of super nutrients. I'm sure you can literally find and eat something red, orange, yellow, green, blue, indigo and yes, even violet!

Try to go for more vegetables than fruit, as some fruits are quite high in sugar. However much you eat, think about getting a nice mix, and always have your fruit *with* meals (I'm assuming that you wouldn't eat vegetables as a snack!). **Eat a rainbow of plants**.

Juices and smoothies may contain natural ingredients, but they're concentrated in a way that a cavewoman just couldn't rustle up! If you have them from time to time, think about them *as a meal*, or have them *with* meals.

Eating vegetables and fruits makes two things happen. Firstly, you get tiny nutrients that allow your body to work properly, and that includes burning body fat correctly. And secondly, they make eating worse food choices less likely.

5 – SEE HEAVY METAL THREE TIMES PER MONTH

For years, for way too long, training with weights has been viewed as something for the boys. The truth is, it's more important for girls to hit the iron. It builds muscle, bone, shape, strength, firmness, carb control, and *confidence*.

It's so important, that I believe three times per month, you must find a way to visit a gym and have a long workout, just doing weights. Why a gym? You need everything in place to work out hard, safely, and yet have some fun.

If you're scared of going to a gym because of how you feel about your image, don't give up on the idea easily. Find somewhere quiet, or pretty much anywhere you can feel comfortable. **This is your life**. Don't hide away forever.

You don't have to join a gym, as most places will let you pay for a guest workout. Make a morning or afternoon or evening out of it. Train like a guy who is desperate to get the girls! If you need help, get someone to show you around a few times.

If you truly can't stand the thought of a gym, maybe try some classes. Circuit training, Pilates and yoga are all good if they're tough enough. And if that's too much, buy some dumbbells and do something at home. Just do something!

By training your muscles hard at least three times a month, you'll keep your muscle mass where it needs to be, and boost lots of good chemicals. Everyone can do it. **Give your muscles a hard time three times a month**. It'll give you OMGs for life.

And it won't just improve your muscles or level of body fat. The boost from weights is complex, and sends out chemical waves all over your body. Even your skin, hair and nails will improve. We are *all* meant to be strong creatures!

6 – DREAM OF BEING SKINNY

Getting a great sleep is like doing a high-five with your body and brain each night! It says, 'good job, let's do it again tomorrow'. Sleep resets all good chemicals and gives major things like muscles and hormones a chance to rest.

And it's not just about having a long time in bed. The quality of your sleep, that is, how *deep* you sleep, makes a difference in how much growth hormone you produce. That's our main chemical which pretty much makes everything better.

In terms of just being skinny, sleep is important because it boosts your thyroid. That's a hormone that sets the speed of your metabolism. And simply, the rate of your metabolism is the rate at which your body uses energy (calories!).

And even if you are *just* thinking about the outside stuff, like your skin, hair and nails, it's worth remembering that it's during sleep, they get a free makeover! **Sleep in some ways is about *doing nothing*, so do nothing *well*.**

7 – EAT CARBS LIKE A CAVEWOMAN

Right back at the start, I told you that I didn't want you to obsess over labels, count calories, or be scared of fat. Our cave ancestors never did that. The thing is, we don't really live in caves any more. We live in caves on top of caves!

We live in a *modern* world. Some of that's great, and some of it is just too much. Our farming produces too much. The biggest *too much* category, is carbs. And it's become almost impossible to stop them being space invaders in our caves!

But we're smart. We have the knowledge to see them hiding and lurking where we'd least expect. Protein takes care of itself, fat too, and fruit and veg rarely need mentioning. But carbs are naughty nippers, and you've got to keep an eye on them!

Even if you pick the healthiest carbs, too many will make it difficult to stay skinny. Our genes are just too ancient to deal with the products of modern farming. And if you don't respect your genes, the carbs will ruin your jeans!

So, every so often, take a sneak at your source of carbs in a meal. Nothing else, just how many grams you're eating at a sitting. Don't bother counting what's in your vegetables, but **avoid going over 40 grams of carbs per meal**.

This is easily enough for 99% of humans. If you're pregnant or a serious athlete (or, a pregnant serious athlete!), you may need more. But for the massive majority, that's the skinny majority, 40g per meal is enough for brain and muscles to be happy.

I'm not expecting you to look at labels all the time. As I said, every so often, check them out. If you're eating 100g of carbs per meal, cut back! But say you're eating 20g and still feeling good, don't raise it. **40g of carbs per meal is a limit, not a target!**

And if you're out in the wilderness, remember that the space of four *iPhones* or *Blackberrys* represents the maximum amount of carbs that you want to stick to. The main thing is that carbs must never crowd out protein!

And remember, we don't need carbs. We need protein. We need fat. We need vitamins, minerals and nutrients. We need oxygen. We need daylight. We need to stay still (sleep). We need to move (move!). **But we don't need carbs**.

Of course, you'll eat some. And yeah, they're tasty! Without a doubt, life must be fun. The thing is to balance all of this, against how being a less-than-perfect you *feels*. Find the balance. It's extremely personal, but you can find it.

If you need to drop a few pounds for a special occasion, check out your carb quality. Avoid *the fast and the furious*. Sidestep liquid carbs, low-fiber foods, and all those with 'sugar' or 'ose' in the first 3 ingredients. **Keep your friends close and your carbs closer**.

There you have it. 7 things that will look after you, if you look after them. They're not difficult, and with a splash of habit, they'll melt into your days, months and years without you blinking. But what about all the other stuff in the book?

Well, just because you reach the end of a book, it doesn't mean that the techniques are done. If you feel like you need a boost, and are ready for it, why not try a month of *skinny dipping?* You make the rules. Make good ideas *yours.* Work it, own it!

If your routine isn't satisfying you, make sure that you don't do what most humans do: *make clumsy changes.* The so-called phenomenon of yo-yo dieting is one example of this, and it never works. So, what's the solution if fumbling back and forth doesn't get results?

In my experience, for truly breathtaking success, you need to learn a forgotten skill. You need to become masterful at *tweaking.* Tweaking is the art of making delicate, light, on the surface adjustments, and yet being able to sense when going much deeper is needed, and getting stuck in.

There's no easy way to end this book. It might feel like I've held your hand for ages and then suddenly snatched it away. I had to do it. As they never say in slushy movies, *it's not me, it's you!* What are *you* waiting for?

GET THE SKINNY ON...

OMG 6 Never munch without moving first

OMG 5 Eat 3 meals per day and kick snacks to the curb

OMG 4 Fill half of your plate with a source of mostly protein

OMG 3 Eat a colorful mix of fruit and veg every day

OMG 2 Do a tough weights workout 3 times per month

OMG 1 Sleep deep every night and wake when you want to

OMG ! Never eat more than 40 grams of pure carbs per meal (4 smartphones!)

THE JOY OF SIX

What, you're still *here*? As in, not *out of here* doing the business. Why not? Stand up, run, scream, do something! It's okay, I'm joking. If you're anything like me, you'll need a final nudge in the right direction.

This book was never about scaring you (not even the stuff in the tub), but always about empowerment (even the stuff in the tub). In yet another nutshell, this book, getting healthy, wearing skinnier jeans, and even your life itself, is about *joy*.

That means, take a look at what I've written here, and play with it. Approach your plan with confidence and fun, and don't *ever* (translation: **ever**) beat yourself up for having a bad week.

52 bad weeks in a row becomes a bad year, but *one* bad week? It's a blip! Great plans get ruined if there's too much pressure to do them perfectly. Even Mother Nature isn't perfect (have you ever seen a duck-billed platypus? *Google* it.).

If you make *one* good improvement during a week, you're still moving faster than those sitting on the couch. Got that? Doh! **If you make *one* good improvement during a week, you're still moving faster than those sitting on the couch!**

And never forget perhaps the most important thing about any plan: *you* are the one doing it! That makes *you* the boss. *You* run

Insert-Your-Name-Here LLC. **You** are powerful. Make smart daily decisions and make your body smash the Fortune 500.

Okay, first up, here's how an average **day** flows in sequence:

Upon waking	Have a tall glass of water.
	Run the bath (or put the shower on).
	Get some black coffee ready (or lay out caffeine pills!).
Hit the bathroom	Check the temperature's not too cold.
	Start your timer, and step in!
	When the timer's up, get out, and get dressed.
Drink up	Get that coffee down you!
Hunt	Get moving (*anything* that's enjoyable)!
	Don't think about speed, just aim to keep moving.
	If you don't hit your goal, keep calm, it's just a day.
Wait	Finish your moving, make a mental note of the time.
	Wait at least 60 minutes until you eat something.
	As you get comfortable, *build up* to a 180 minute gap.

Breakfast	You get to eat breakfast at last (about 'lunch time' for many)!
	Find a big chunk of protein to dominate your plate.
	If you like fruit, have some at this meal.
Hunt again	Before your second meal, get moving (it *won't* take long).
	Remember, movement is movement, find a way.
Wait again	Leave a small gap (15 to 30 minutes) until you eat.
Second meal	This will be about 3 to 5 hours after your 'breakfast'.
	Keep the protein up, and drink some green tea if you can.
Evening hunt	Before your traditional last evening meal, move some more.
	Try some fun form of movement (if you're getting bored!).
Wait (yet) again	Leaving a 15 minute gap after this last POM session is crucial.
Final meal	This will also be 3 to 5 hours after your second meal.
	Try to avoid fruit in this meal if possible.

Stick to those carb limits (it'll make tomorrow easier).

Sleep   Get some!

Make sure that final meal isn't too close to bed time.

Everyone is different, even identical twins. So, rather than be totally exact about how you *must* do things, here are some **key thoughts** to help you focus on what's important, and navigate your way through the six weeks.

These key thoughts aren't random by the way. They're entirely logical. By building on each *thought*, they'll gradually overlap each other until you reach a point where every key change is being made *at once*. Doing it like this feels effortless.

WEEK 1 KEY THOUGHT: start living off yourself

Your first week will be a *transition*. If you're reading this book, it's likely that you're coming from a place of frustration, and a desire to change. Remind yourself of those two things often, because this week is one of the toughest.

The most important thing during this first week is to start the shift from living constantly *on* food, to living *off* you. The best way of doing this is to move in the morning. If you can't face the baths, at least get moving first thing.

253

WEEK 2 KEY THOUGHT: keep the protein up and love the gap

The second week of any plan can be difficult. The boost of motivation from the first few days is often slipping, and now you're faced with the cold reality of hard work. In fact, it *doesn't* need to be hard work. It can, be easy.

Controlling your appetite is going to be crucial at this stage. Make it an absolute priority to fill half of every meal's plate with protein. Doing this will allow you to go for longer between meals, and help build on the first week's changes.

WEEK 3 KEY THOUGHT: stop creeping over those carb limits

Okay, now it's getting tough! By now, you ideally will have a regular morning pattern of waking up and moving (and ideally, doing the Skinny Dipping before it). Carbs are the test of *every* diet, so it's time to start giving them proper attention.

Spend some time this week, looking at labels. Yes, it *is* boring! And yes, it *is* important. Get *under* those carb limits, and by the end of this third week, your food cravings and entire physiology would have started to change for good.

WEEK 4 KEY THOUGHT: don't lose what you have

Most people who try 'diet' books, concentrate just on food, and then spend some time on what's traditionally known as 'cardio' (I still won't mention the "E" word!). About 4 weeks in, is when muscle loss starts to happen. This must be prevented.

Your muscles are your friendly furnaces that burn energy all day long. Keep the furnaces firing by hitting the weights, or doing a gym studio class that really challenges your muscles. Your metabolism is *depending* on you to do this.

WEEK 5 KEY THOUGHT: get precise

If you haven't been doing it already (or have perhaps forgotten), there are lots of things within food that make progress more difficult. Excess added sugars, certain kinds of fat, and marketing tricks played by stores can be a minefield.

By now, you're moving early, controlling your appetite, leaving gaps, and preserving your muscle. Eliminate the tiny gremlins such as foods with "ose" on the label, hydrogenated fats and be especially wary of foods marked "healthy".

WEEK 6 KEY THOUGHT: keep your eye on the prize

As we approach a finish line, whether it's a turn in the road, or literally, a finishing tape on the track, we tend to relax. When it comes to health, this isn't ideal. Six weeks was a start, but it's *not* the final destination.

Start to plan how you can take these new changes forward, rather than start to plan what you'll do "once I finish". Adapt them as necessary, so that they continue beyond the six weeks, and blend in so that you hardly notice.

WEEK 7 & KEY THOUGHTS FOR LIFE:

Well, that's up to you! Seriously, by this point, your body will have changed dramatically, even if you haven't seen all the outside changes you imagined. I can **assure** you, good stuff will be going on inside.

If you still feel like you're on a plan at this point, something's up. Get out your hammer and chisel, and sculpt away at what you've learned until it fits *your* life. Good health isn't just a short-term concept. Make it work permanently.

For the six weeks itself, it can be nice to follow guidelines though, and just in case you've forgotten who you are, I've put a reminder below. As I said way back, try not to chop and change between the levels (but do if you really *have* to).

WAVE, BLAZE & QUAKE SPECIFIC GUIDELINES

Skinny Dipping (*never* get into water that's below 15 degrees Celsius!)

Wave   Stand for 2 minutes
            Sit for 8 minutes

Blaze   Stand for 2 minutes
            Sit for 3 minutes
            Lay for 5 minutes

Quake   Stand for 2 minutes
            Sit for 3 minutes
            Lay for 10 minutes

Hunt & Wait (pick *any* form of movement you like, and wait after!)

Wave   POM 1 - 30 minutes upon waking (+ 60 to 180 minutes before food)
              POM 2 - 15 minutes before 2nd meal (+ 15 minutes wait before food)
              POM 3 - 15 minutes before 3rd meal (+ 15 minutes wait before food)

Blaze   POM 1 - 45 minutes upon waking (+ 60 to 180 minutes before food)
              POM 2 - 15 minutes before 2nd meal (+ 30 minutes wait before food)
              POM 3 - 15 minutes before 3rd meal (+ 15 minutes wait before food)

Quake   POM 1 - 45 minutes upon waking (+ 60 to 180 minutes before food)
              POM 2 - 30 minutes before 2nd meal (+ 30 minutes wait before food)
              POM 3 - 15 minutes before 3rd meal (+ 15 minutes wait before food)

Carbs (limits *not* targets!)

Wave   120 grams per day (roughly 3 meals of 40 grams per meal)

Blaze   90 grams per day (roughly 3 meals of 30 grams per meal)

Quake	60 grams per day (roughly 3 meals of 20 grams per meal)

Fruits (avoid all dried fruits!)

Wave	3 pieces maximum per day (one per meal)
Blaze	2 pieces maximum per day (avoid fruit in your final meal)
Quake	1 piece maximum per day (have that in your first meal)

THE FIRST CHAPTER

Yes, you've done it, you've crossed the I – finish line – I!
Really well done. And now that you have finished, it's time to
start! All the knowledge in the world is *junk* if it just sits in the
back of that giant drawer known as your brain!

There maybe times when you've struggled to understand what
you've read. **Don't beat yourself up**. It's so important to have
some love for yourself. Do this for me: shut your eyes and imagine you're looking after someone's new baby.

The baby's walking. Oops, they fell. Are you shouting at them?
I doubt it. Oops, they - did - it - again. Still not shouting? Of
course not! You accept that it takes time for a baby to learn how
to walk. It takes time for you to master new skills too. And once
you do, they're with you for life. So, be cool.

Listen to me, listen out for new ideas, but listen to you also.
Become the expert. **Everyone can at least become an expert
on themselves!** Once you do that, you'll be a big step closer to
owning something that will give you the *ultimate* personality.

Confidence. It's a word that we hear a lot, but some words never
work on paper, and that's one of them. Because confidence is a
feeling. And what a feeling it is! With confidence, **you** have the
power to do anything.

As the world grows bigger, and sometimes scarier, you'll need something to keep you strong. That something is confidence. And a ridiculously big chunk of that comes from how you see yourself.

This isn't just a diet book. It's a confidence book. Never underestimate the power of confidence. Find it, keep it, and above all, use it to have a fantastic life. Thanks for sharing the journey. See you at the top.

GET THE SKINNY ON...

OMG 6 Need more? veniceafulton.com

OMG 5 Need free support? mysixweeks.com

OMG 4 Need to show off? facebook.com/omgdiet

OMG 3 Need to Tweet me something? @veniceafulton

OMG 2 Need to use your Blackberry instead of measuring carbs with it?

OMG 1 Need another excuse to keep reading stuff, then look below

OMG ! Turn off your laptop, turn on your neck-top, and go get your OMGs!

WHO TOLD YOU THAT?

There are times in life, when no one will believe you. And, there will be times in life when you don't believe others. Perhaps you *still* don't believe me? Good! Because that means like all clever creatures, you deserve **proof**.

Proof saves us from embarrassment, proof saves us from wasting time, and proof even saves us from being squished when Laura the Lemming screams 'JUMP OFF THE CLIFF'! Scientists call proof *evidence based thinking*.

Once you find *evidence*, you need to decide what to do with it. That's **use it or move it**. If you don't do anything, you'll end up in a ghost town called *Nowhere*. That's the place where most scientists live.

Scientists often wait years before they decide what to do with research. Each breakthrough is treated like a tiny dot on a giant dot-to-dot picture. And to be fair, geeks can afford to relax. After all, lab coats are great at hiding thighs of any size!

For most of us, there's no time to be wishy-washy. Instead, **it is necessary to join the dots and make sense of the bigger picture, even before all the dots have arrived.** Science calls this 'guesswork'. I call it 'I get the picture, let's give it a go'!

The truth is, everything is guesswork in some sense. Why? Because the fact is, *facts don't exist*. **All we have are educated guesses**. When we have enough guesses, we join them together and call it a *fact*.

In the future, some facts in this book may get replaced by newer ones. Perhaps we'll invent drugs or therapies that make getting an OMG body as simple as taking a pill. Until then, we have to do the best with what we know.

I've got some of the best things that I know *work* and put them here. It's a great place to start. I've changed the research titles to help explain what they're talking about. If you have access to the internet, you're just a click away. Everything is:

- In peer (geek) reviewed scientific journals

- Published in the 21st century (i.e. discovered after 2000)

- Researched using humans (and that means no monkeys either!)

- Available at **pubmed.gov** (type in the **PubMed ID** to find the study)

Why your doctor might not be an expert on diet

American Journal of Clinical Nutrition in 2006

PubMed ID 16600952

Losing weight is related to improving the quality of life in general

Eating Behaviors in 2009

PubMed ID 19447349

Even losing less than 5% of bodyweight improves how dynamic we feel

Health and Quality of Life Outcomes in 2006

PubMed ID 16846509

Trust yourself, because others telling you what to do can make things worse

Social Science and Medicine in 2010

PubMed ID 19944507

Body Mass Index (BMI) isn't useful for most people

International Journal of Obesity in 2008

PubMed ID 18283284

Body Mass Index (BMI) isn't useful for detecting heart disease

European Heart Journal in 2007

PubMed ID 17626030

Body Mass Index (BMI) is mentally too harsh or too soothing to help anyone

Australian and New Zealand Journal of Psychiatry in 2009

PubMed ID 19530022

BMI, tape measures and body fat percentages could all be ineffective

American Journal of Clinical Nutrition in 2009

PubMed ID 19116329

Listening to the media isn't the smartest way to decide how you must look

Pediatrics in 2007

PubMed ID 17200254

If you lose weight too fast, you could shrink organs and that reduces metabolism

American Journal of Clinical Nutrition in 2009

PubMed ID 19710198

Bulimia messes with how the body deals with food, making it better at getting fat

American Journal of Nutrition in 2005

PubMed ID 16093401

In most people with eating disorders, it's simply not about being skinny

The International Journal of Eating Disorders in 2002

PubMed ID 12386908

Drugs probably won't cure you of eating disorders

International Journal of Neuropsychopharmacology in 2012

PubMed ID 21439105

If you have an eating disorder, helping yourself could be the best strategy

International Journal of Eating Disorders in 2004

PubMed ID 15101068

Weighing yourself is associated with successful weight loss

Journal of the American Dietetic Association in 2011

PubMed ID 21185970

The scales in your doctor's surgery or gym are probably inaccurate

Public Health Reports (Washington DC) in 2005

PubMed ID 16134566

Skipping breakfast can make people moan, but they still don't overeat later

American Journal of Clinical Nutrition in 2011

PubMed ID 21084650

Breakfast skipping doesn't actually reduce concentration

Journal of Developmental and Behavioral Pediatrics in 2012

PubMed ID 22218013

If you breakfast like a king, you'll probably end up eating like one all day

Nutrition Journal in 2011

PubMed ID 21241465

Young overweight kids who skip breakfast lose weight, but normal ones don't

International Journal of Obesity and Related Metabolic Disorders in 2003

PubMed ID 14513075

Some people are just starting to study breakfast skipping

Trials in 2011

PubMed ID 21740575

BAT exists in humans, and the more you have, the better

PLoS One (Public Library of Science) in 2011

PubMed ID 21390318

A cold water bathing suit increased body fat fuel burning by 376%

Journal of Applied Physiology in 2002

PubMed ID 12070189

BAT exists in adults and helps them burn fat when it's cold

The Journal of Clinical Investigation in 2012

PubMed ID 22269323

Coffee and green tea combined cause sustained and powerful fat loss

Obesity Reviews in 2011

PubMed ID 21366839

Multiple movement sessions beat moving the same amount all in one go

Journal of Applied Physiology in 2007

PubMed ID 17317872

Move more muscle at any one time (e.g. run vs. cycle) and you'll burn more fat

Metabolism in 2003

PubMed ID 12800102

Movement is more effective for losing body fat than cutting back on food

The Journal of Nutritional Biochemistry in 2003

PubMed ID 14505816

Moving slow or fast makes no difference when it comes to shrinking your belly

American Journal of Clinical Nutrition in 2009

PubMed ID 19211823

Just moving around keeps the resting metabolic rate stoked up

Journal of the American Dietetic Association in 2001

PubMed ID 11678489

If you walk or run, you'll burn calories, but running will make you hungrier

American Journal of Clinical Nutrition in 2004

PubMed ID 15531670

Your body will stay skinnier if you ignore what day of the week it is

International Journal of Obesity and Related Metabolic Disorders in 2004

PubMed ID 14647183

To beat appetite, a protein-rich first meal helps your brain combat food cravings

Obesity in 2011

PubMed ID 21546927

Eating 6 times per day doesn't make you skinnier than eating 3 times per day

British Journal of Nutrition in 2011

PubMed ID 19943985

Snacks might contain healthy nutrients, but they're not healthy overall

Journal of the American Dietetic Association in 2011

PubMed ID 22117666

Fatter people tend to snack more

International Journal of Obesity in 2005

PubMed ID 15809664

Increased dietary protein leads to reduced appetite even when food is limitless

American Journal of Clinical Nutrition in 2008

PubMed ID 18469287

If you prioritize good quality protein, you're likely to have a skinnier middle

Nutrition and Metabolism in 2012

PubMed ID 22284338

Protein reduces appetite more than fat and carbs, and our brain controls that

Current Opinion in Clinical Nutrition and Metabolic Care in 2009

PubMed ID 19057188

Wherever there's western food, there's trouble

Journal of Obesity in 2012

PubMed ID 22235369

You'll burn less fat if you eat a high-carb diet

American Journal of Clinical Nutrition in 2008

PubMed ID 18400703

The carb to fat ratio in the diet heavily influences how much body fat you make

The Proceedings of the Nutrition Society in 2002

PubMed 12133211

In some people, it's just total carbs that determines how fat they'll be

Journal of the American Dietetic Association in 2007

PubMed ID 17904937

Soft drinks could mean you're eating more junk, but you still might be skinny

Journal of Nutrition in 2012

PubMed ID 22223568

For most people, liquid carbs are likely to make you take in too much energy

American Journal of Clinical Nutrition in 2012

PubMed ID 22258267

Solid food keeps hunger controlled longer than softer food with the same calories

Journal of the American Dietetic Association in 2008

PubMed ID 18589034

The thickness of a food is linked to how happy it makes you feel after eating it

Journal of Nutrition in 2009

PubMed ID 19176745

Higher levels of fructose will make your belly stick out, even if you're young

Journal of Nutrition in 2012

PubMed ID 22190023

Adding fructose to meals can make them go from bad to worse

Proceedings of the National Academy of Sciences of the USA in 2012

PubMed ID 22315413

Eating or drinking a source of fructose before walking, reduces body fat burning

European Journal of Applied Physiology in 2011

PubMed ID 22081046

Dietary fat has finally been cleared of the crime it didn't commit

Cochrane Database of Systematic Reviews in 2008

PubMed ID 18646093

People on lower carb diets do better than those on low-fat diets

Annals of Internal Medicine in 2004

PubMed ID 15148064

If you're young and heavy, getting more Omega 3 fats could help you get skinny

Archives of Medical Research in 2011

PubMed ID 22136960

6 weeks of fish oil could helps you lose a pound of fat and gain a pound of muscle

Journal of the International Society of Sports Nutrition in 2010

PubMed ID 20932294

Having carbs close to movement stops body fat loss and turns off caveman genes

American Journal of Physiology, Endocrinology and Metabolism in 2005

PubMed ID 16030063

Gaps between moving and eating can increase body fat burning

Nutrition in 2004

PubMed ID 15212756

Pumping iron will help stop you losing muscle when you're changing your diet

Obesity in 2009

PubMed ID 19247271

Having more muscle means you'll be burning more calories all the time

Obesity Reviews in 2002

PubMed ID 12120418

Training with weights improves how insulin works, even in older people

Journal of the American Geriatrics Society in 2001

PubMed ID 11300234

Strength training is suitable and safe for young children and teens

Journal of the American Academy of Orthopaedic Surgeons in 2001

PubMed ID 11174161

Hitting the weights will stop excess carbs from hitting your body hard

Diabetes in 2004

PubMed ID 14747278

Weights combined with some impact movement increases female bone strength

Journal of Bone and Mineral Metabolism in 2010

PubMed ID 20013013

Blowing up balloons isn't a party trick and helps posture and your midsection

North American Journal of Sports Physical Therapy in 2010

PubMed ID 21589673

Stress makes you eat junk, and get a big belly

Psychoneuroendocrinology in 2011

PubMed ID 21906885

Gift wrapping your organs in visceral fat can be damaging for health

Circulation in 2007

PubMed ID 17576866

Visceral fat causes higher levels of inflammation than fat just under the skin

Internal Medicine in 2011

PubMed ID 22082888

If you're fat, and have lots of inflammation, consuming Omega 3 fat will help

British Journal of Nutrition in 2011

PubMed ID 22133051

Deep fat is linked to greater problems with arthritis and heart disease

Autoimmunity Reviews in 2011

PubMed ID 21539940

Most carbs will make you crave them again and again

Current Neuropharmacology in 2011

PubMed ID 22131945

Junk food really is addictive

Current Drug Abuse Reviews in 2011

PubMed ID 21999689

Stress that keeps you up will make you start craving the worst kind of food

Journal of Sleep Research in 2010

PubMed ID 20545838

If you want a boost of growth hormone from movement, don't drink alcohol

Neuro Endocrinology Letters in 2007

PubMed ID 17435673

If you sleep less than normal, you'll eat more and probably move about less

American Journal of Clinical Nutrition in 2011

PubMed ID 21715510

Even if you're healthy, one night's bad sleep ruins how your body processes food

Journal of Clinical Endocrinology and Metabolism in 2010

PubMed ID 20371664

A lack of sleep will increase your appetite, and make food less satisfying

Annals of the New York Academy of Sciences in 2008

PubMed ID 18591489

If you're moving about less today, it could be because you slept less last night

American Journal of Clinical Nutrition in 2011

PubMed ID 21471283

Don't eat too close to bedtime, or you'll mess up your hormones

Molecular and Cellular Endocrinology in 2012

PubMed ID 21939733

If you don't sleep well tonight, you're weakening your skin

Brain, Behavior and Immunity in 2009

PubMed ID 19523511

If you're young and don't sleep much, you'll eat more, move less, and be fat

International Journal of Obesity in 2011

PubMed ID 21792170

Snacks soon become more common than meals in those who don't sleep much

American Journal of Clinical Nutrition in 2009

PubMed ID 19056602

Using water at meals might help you control your appetite

Nutrition Reviews in 2010

PubMed ID 20796216

Artificial sweeteners may not be sweet and innocent in terms of fat loss

The Yale Journal of Biology and Medicine in 2010

PubMed ID 20589192

If you're not properly hydrated, you might not boost helpful growth hormone

European Journal of Endocrinology in 2001

PubMed ID 11581003

Humans know how to drink enough water

Sports Medicine in 2007

PubMed ID 17465636

If you keep your blood sugar high all the time, you'll have older looking skin

Age in 2011

PubMed ID 22102339

Massaging thighs and lymphatic drainage reduces cellulite

Journal of the European Academy of Dermatology and Venereology in 2010

PubMed ID 19627407

By wobbling skin with an acoustic wave, you boost collagen and reduce cellulite

Aesthetic Surgery Journal in 2008

PubMed ID 19083577

Green tea reduces appetite and increases the use of body fat as a fuel

The Journal of Nutritional Biochemistry in 2011

PubMed ID 21115335

Green tea makes you lose more belly fat when you're moving around

The Journal of Nutrition in 2009

PubMed ID 19074207

Don't believe the hype, as not all food labels are there to serve you

Nutrition Reviews in 2010

PubMed ID 20883420

Organic food doesn't mean that it's likely to keep you skinny

International Journal of Food Sciences and Nutrition in 2003

PubMed ID 12907407

Organic food still doesn't mean that it's safe

Critical Reviews in Food Science and Nutrition in 2006

PubMed ID 16403682

Stores use marketing that helps you get fatter

Annual Review of Public Health in 2011

PubMed ID 21219166

Rotating your fruit and vegetables is healthy and can help prevent cancers

Nutrition and Cancer in 2004

PubMed ID 15231448

Mixing up your vegetable matter could help stop you having heart disease

Annals of Internal Medicine in 2001

PubMed ID 11412050

High intakes of vegetables and fruit are linked to superior weight loss

Nutrition Research in 2008

PubMed ID 19083413

It's easier to get a bigger butt, if you choose a bigger portion

American Journal of Clinical Nutrition in 2002

PubMed ID 12450884

Even chefs admit how the size of their portion affects your love of their food

Obesity in 2007

PubMed ID 17712127

Even if you believe in calories, foods and restaurants can be hugely inaccurate

Journal of the American Dietetic Association in 2011

PubMed ID 20102837

Diets that just focus on low-calories can raise inflammatory cortisol

Psychosomatic Medicine in 2010

PubMed ID 20368473

Calories aren't always what they say they are, so why bother

Journal of the International Society of Sports Nutrition in 2004

PubMed ID 18500946

VISIT VENICE

Using a cheeky mix of science, psychology and uncommon sense, Venice A. Fulton has helped many humans and selected pets get skinny fast. Most have enjoyed working with Venice, although one dog barked about the cold baths.

A former writer for *Celebrity Bodies* magazine (it did exist), Venice knows all about the importance of speed in the transformation process. In fact, *Six Weeks to OMG* was written during an elevator journey.

Venice A. Fulton is currently on the run from the world's biggest cereal companies, who want to delete the book's section on skipping breakfast. Venice sometimes hides in London, England. Don't tell them.

THANKS

Thanks to Robert Noyce and Jack Kilby, inventors of the microchip, who made our modern world possible. Thanks to Bill Gates, who cooked their chips into a practical meal. Thanks to Tim Berners-Lee, who used Bill's dish to serve up the internet. And thanks to Steve Jobs, who made everything digital taste cool.

Thanks to Jeff Bezos, founder of Amazon, and JK Rowling, creator of Harry Potter, who between them have kept books in our hearts, and more importantly, in our hands.

Thanks to the superbly named, Marshall Brain, founder of How Stuff Works, who encouraged me, and underlined my belief in creating intellectual property.

Thanks to Mark Twain. You're perhaps the most inspiring dead guy I know. Apologies for not using your quote about health books. Save me a seat in the naughty corner.

Thanks to CJ Allan of CJ's Easy As Pie site. When I was really stuck in the technical mud, you came along with a mental 4x4 and dug me out. Much respect.

Thanks to Michael Colgan, PhD of The Colgan Institute. Your insights into nutrition are outstanding. If I've stolen any of your smartness, I've stolen from the best.

Thanks to Sarah Ballard, who took a chance on me at United Agents in London. Despite looking after the Booker Prize winner, she made time to fit in something with OMG in the title. Project Richmond is coming soon.

Thanks to Jessica Craig at United Agents, who displays a particular genius in generating a passport for the book, and getting it across borders into places I've yet heard of. How do you say OMG in Mandarin?

Thanks to Katy Follain at Penguin, my super calm and super talented editor. The thought of someone editing my work was quite scary, until I met you. You're a magic elf that creeps down in the night, and fixes everything by morning.

Thanks to Louise Moore at Penguin, who took an innocent little Word file, and turned it into paper across the globe. They say it takes talent to spot talent, but I just blame sheer good luck for bumping into you.

Thanks to everyone else at Penguin. Anyone who watches wildlife programs will know how brilliant penguins are. They're funny, smart, tough, and they have a real sense of family. They even love cold baths! It's a perfect match.

Thanks to Diana Baroni, Matthew Ballast and Jamie Raab, my wonderful publishing triumvirate at Grand Central in New York. Their low-key style almost had me fooled, but when it came down to it, that was merely a sign of three extremely cool and capable heads.

Thanks to David Young, CEO of Hachette, who managed to find my book floating along the electronic ether. While many companies would be sitting back on their vampire trilogy laurels, David opted to take a big bite into a health book.

Thanks to my super US agent, Richard Pine of InkWell Management in NY. His track record of bestsellers speaks for itself, but nothing prepared me for his bestselling personality. Every email and call is an education.

Thanks to Michael Carlisle at InkWell Management in NY, who despite being an American, displays more European finesse than me. Your heartfelt advice will always stick with me.

Thanks to Kim Witherspoon, and the rest of the team at Ink-Well Management, who have made me feel at home, despite being thousands of miles away from a proper cup of tea.

Thanks to Anna Freedman, a stranger who shrunk the world by appearing in the library one day, at the same table, and happened to be writing a diet book. Bizarre! Can't wait.

Thanks to Maria Smith, for being a good friend, and for keeping me on track at tough times.

Thanks to Uzo Ehiogu, another great friend, who inspired me to write before I knew I could. Write something yourself now, because your scientific brain has so much to offer.

Thanks to Duncan Meadows, whose monotone advice to "get it done" often rung like an annoying woodpecker in my ears.

Thanks to Sab Sayed, whose "let's see" got me keen to do exactly that.

Thanks to Tony Nath, whose constant "have you done it yet?", can now be answered: DONE IT!

Thanks to the building, the staff and the fellow users of Church End library in Finchley, London, where this book was dreamt up, written, and may even be read. A library is a home of ideas, and you made it a very welcoming home.

Thanks to my 12 year old nephew Cameron, who has offered to promote this book to every girl he knows. I hope you know a few million.

Thanks to Rob Skinner, whose rebellious and philosophical ways helped set the cheeky tone to which this book whistles. If I get in trouble, I'm pointing at you!

Thanks to Mark Woollard, whose smart questions kept me on my toes like a Meerkat. Thanks to Jenny Woollard, whose intelligent and gentle reminder of why I was writing echoed in my mind. Thanks to both of you for making a certain Bella.

And finally, thanks to the rest of my family, who have apparently put up with me since I was born.

The best way to predict the future, is to invent it.

Fortune Cookie (high carb)